The Power of Champions
Helping Readers Find Their Absolute Physical Best

By Phil Kaplan & the Fitness Champions

Published by:
     Great Atlantic Publishing Group
     1304 SW 160th Avenue #337
     Sunrise, FL 33326

The illustrations in the Introduction were provided by and are the copyrighted property of:
VHI Inc., P.O. Box 44646, Tacoma, WA 98444, 253-536-4922.

Distributed in the U.S. by the American Association of Personal Trainers (AAPT)
3132 Fortune Way, #D-1, Wellington, FL 33414

Library of Congress Control Number: 2004101880
Library of Congress Cataloging in Publication Data
Kaplan, Phil
     The Power of Champions
     Helping Readers Find Their Absolute Physical Best
     ISBN 1-887463097
     1. Physical Fitness   2. Health   3. Nutrition   I. Title
     II. Title: The Power of Champions

Additional copies of this book may be purchased for $24.99 plus
$4.00 shipping and handling from:
   AAPT
   3132 Fortune Way, #D-1
   Wellington, Florida 33414
   888-311-2278

Contents

SECTION FIVE
The Heart of A Champion 143

SECTION SIX
Eat Like a Champion 155

SECTION SEVEN
Perform Like a Champion 193

SECTION EIGHT
Champions Break Barriers! 209

SECTION NINE
Champion "Down Time" 229

How *The Power of Champions* Came to Be

Phil Kaplan, author of <u>The Best You've Ever Been</u> and host of the ***Mind & Muscle Fitness Hour Radio Show***, is a renowned fitness professional who has been changing bodies and lives for over two decades.

In 2003, Phil accepted a position as President of the American Association of Personal Trainers (AAPT) with one primary stipulation. He was going to handpick the premier members of this organization and create a respected and credible group of fitness professionals, a group that can stand as a model of Personal Training Excellence.

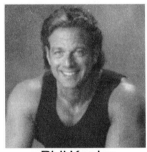

Phil Kaplan

"As I began to survey the landscape, to really explore the field of trainers in search of the true cream of the crop, I was both dismayed and excited. I was dismayed by the lack of professionalism in a field built upon such a noble foundation as health and fitness, but as I came in contact with the true leaders, with the members of the ground army who were making a difference on a daily basis, I realized a true core of professionals exist. As the fitness-wanting public has embarked upon a fruitless search in quest of a vehicle for positive physical change, people are directed via the media to attempt to change with what I call ineffective technologies. While tummy reducers, fat-burning pills, and miracle diets battle for attention, and those who fall for their offerings are the unfortunate victims of the battle, I had identified a gold mine. Every one of the 55 fitness professionals I found to represent the AAPT had an important message to share, a message founded in truth, and if 55 professional voices all band together to help people find the realities behind fitness, weight loss, and physical improvement, "The Power" these "Champions" can deliver would help people cut through the fraud and deception to find true empowerment.

I want to extend my admiration and gratitude to the 55 champions who have worked with me to co-author a book I know will have a dramatic impact upon the health and well being of many, a book that I sincerely hope will begin America and the world on a path toward betterment.

A special thank you to Debbie Hickey, Kelli Calabrese and Ray Simmons who all bought into the vision and worked together to turn the vision into reality. Together we and the 55 Champions join in a single wish. We look to the future with the hope that The Power of Champions *is a power acquired by all who stand to benefit."*

INTRODUCTION: Get Up!

By Phil Kaplan

If you're sitting or lying down, I'm going to ask you to stand up. Yes, right now. Take the book with you, and just get up on your feet. Go ahead and stand up.

Are you on your feet? If you are, then you're to be congratulated. You not only invested in a book, but you actually acted when it asked you to act! I'd love to believe that upon reading the opening words, everyone who opened this book got on their feet, but I know better. Most people didn't.

I KNOW YOU, AND I HOLD THE MAP!

I know you better than you think I do, even if we've never met. For over 20 years people from every walk of life have been walking into my office, visiting with me at my seminars, and have been calling, e-mailing, and reaching out asking me for "the secrets." They may initially appear to have different wants.

Some insist they want to *trim their thighs.*

Others insist they want to *lose weight.*

Some insist that *muscle gain* is the ultimate goal.

Others insist they want to capture that elusive animal called *energy.*

Really what they're asking me for is "the secret to feeling good about themselves." Most of them have been convinced, thanks to years of advertising, marketing, infomercials, twisted research, manipulative conmen, miraculous cellulite cures, and the absurd promises of solutions arriving in little bottles, that there is in fact some magical secret and they set out like a disjointed horde of treasure hunters in search of a great treasure. Like crazed hungry pirates they travel from health food store to health club, from internet offering to sporting goods store, hoping they're zeroing in on the spot marked by the fitness "X." Somewhere along the journey they come to me hoping that I might hold the map that will finally lead them to The Buried Treasure of the Fitness Secret.

Is there a secret? Well, yes, there is, and I do have the map. It's just unfortunate that the true fitness secret has become harder to uncover than the lost treasure of the Incas.

The secret is simple, but unless you're willing to act when I ask you to act, unless you're willing to at least believe in the possibility that this secret may in fact be the treasure, I'll urge you to sit back down, close this book, pick up the phone, and order some bleached and refined flour covered with sodium laden sauce, piled high with extra saturated fat and a heaping helping of preservatives and nitrates. Can I say that in fewer words? Sure. Order a pizza with extra cheese and pepperoni and forget this fitness thing altogether.

At this point you're in one of three situations.

> ***Situation #1:*** You're dialing the number of the local pizza shop. That wouldn't be the ideal situation.

> ***Situation #2:*** If you haven't gone to the phone, you're standing wondering why the nut who conceptualized this book is talking about treasure and making you stand. That's good. That's exactly where I want you to be.

> ***Situation #3:*** You're still sitting or lying down, and still reading.

I'd prefer to eliminate the third group. If you're not on your feet and you're still reading . . . get up!

* * *

OK, now for those who have opted to remain pizza free, at least for the next few minutes (and don't worry, nobody's going to ask you to remain pizza free for any great length of time), I'm going to ask you to do two things, two simple things. Consider them the first two steps toward the treasure.

Breathe deeply, not as you typically do, but take a breath that actually fills your lungs. You'll be surprised how long and deep that breath can be. Then release it slowly and fully. I mean exhale until there's nothing left to exhale, and then, fill your lungs again. Repeat that five times. You feel more alert? More awake? Even slightly energized? That's oxygen doing its thing, and oxygen is a vital part of this process.

This is a little tougher now. Nobody's looking, and if they are, who cares? You're about to get fit while they just sit and stare at you. Let 'em stare. I want you to raise up on your toes as high as you can, as if you're trying to push the ground downward using the balls of your feet. Raise your heels as high as possible and continue the effort for about 2 seconds. Then lower for a count of 3 and do it again, but the second time hold the muscle contraction for 3 seconds. Repeat this rising and lowering for 5 repetitions, increasing the muscle contraction time by 1 second on each consecutive rep, and then relax. You've just stimulated the muscles of your calf.

Now that really was simple, wasn't it? Don't get overly confident. You're not ready to jump on stage and nab the biggest trophy at the next fitness competition that comes to town, at least not yet, but you've experienced the essence of the secret. There are two physical components of physical betterment. Aerobic activity stimulating greater use of oxygen is one, and intentional muscular contraction following a pattern of progressive resistance is the second.

Now you can sit, relax, open up your mind, and prepare to live as the Champions do, with a driving commitment to betterment, one that makes the process of physical change so simple and so rewarding you'll never go back to any other way of life. Who are the Champions? They are the masters of this science of physical change, the individuals who comprise the ground army of fitness truth. They walk the talk and personally live a fitness lifestyle, not because they have to, but because they thoroughly enjoy all the rewards it brings. They are the passion-driven individuals who find a great sense of gratification in helping others master the fitness lifestyle. They have the courage to challenge fitness fraud, the heart required to share their passion and knowledge, and an attitude fired by the ability to empower others. They have the muscle it takes to move figurative mountains, the power required to stimulate action, and the integrity to stay on course and do the right thing, even when that in and of itself is challenging. They have that special something, that optimistic "success at all costs" aura that makes people want to be around them, and they have the unyielding nerve to tell people what they need to hear, even when it isn't what they may want to hear. They are the true Champions of fitness and the co-authors of this book.

I've asked those individuals I feel are making a difference on a daily basis, those who have gone above and beyond the responsibilities of a Personal Fitness Trainer, those who aspire to fitness excellence, to share the information you, the reader, need to take control of the physical structure you live in so you too can live as a Champion.

What Do You Need?

Many infomercials and advertisers will tell you what you need to get fit, and those needs will often come in the form of pills or products with price tags ranging from three easy payments of $12.99 all the way up to three easy payments of $1299. Do you need anything at all? Yes, you do, but what you need cannot be valued with a dollar amount, and in fact, it already exists somewhere within you. You just have to find it.

In order to make a physical change, desire becomes the first necessary requirement. I've never met anyone who told me they "accidentally" got into great shape. No, it always has to begin with a desire, so you need the desire, but desire alone isn't enough. Desire must be accompanied by belief. I don't mean an unwavering belief. I expect there to be some doubt, especially if you've tried to get fit before and failed, but at the very least you have to find a belief in possibility. Many of you may approach this with a "prove it to me" attitude, and that's quite all right. Just realize, unless you believe the change is possible, you're not likely to follow the steps and actions required for it to manifest. Some of you weren't even willing to stand up when I asked! Why? Because you didn't believe it would have any impact. Belief is essential for this process of change. As you read through this book, your belief in possibility will escalate, and when results become apparent, belief will be unshakable, but for now you have to at least buy into the fact that we share the truth, we share a proven technology of change, and we have all come together to lay out a path with the potential to lead right to the ultimate you. Some of you will jump right in, others will tiptoe, but at this point, desire and belief are the requirements.

The Important "Options"

I told you desire and belief are essential. I also told you that you didn't need anything else. That's true, since I know you already have this book and the book shall reveal "the secret" one step at a time. With that said, there are some aids that might make the process simpler, might make the results more dramatic, and might allow you the flexibility to pursue limitless exercise routines.

<u>**Aids for Making the Process a Bit Simpler**</u>

- A couple of pairs of dumbbells or an adjustable dumbbell set
- A good pair of walking or running shoes
- A stability ball
- A heart rate monitor

Identifying and Disempowering Your Enemies

There should, at this point, be a true sense of optimism, a sense that this really is going to work, but before I share the starting exercise routine, the foundational eating strategy, and the advice of the Champions, I feel it important to warn you, enemies are lurking nearby. There are four primary enemies, and if you recognize the damage they can do, you can shut them down completely, destroying any power they have to stand in your way. Here are the four primary enemies:

Television – The television will subtly convince you that you don't have time, but it is the ultimate time parasite. In fact, according to A.C. Neilsen, by the time the average American reaches the age of 65, he or she will have watched the equivalent of 9 years of television!

The Recliner – A conspirator in cahoots with the television, this reclining seat makes you feel so comfortable in the short term, but inactivity, failure to ask the core muscles to support the body, and a firm commitment to a lounging position simply amplify the value of the old adage, "use it or lose it."

The Little Sneaky Devil in Your Head – You know, the voice that shows up to tell you it's better to skip the workout than to get all sweaty. We all have those little competing voices playing against each other. As you begin to recognize your self-talk, you'll also begin to control it, and mentally, quietly, firmly, ask that little discouraging voice to "Please Shut Up!"

The "Yucant" Bug – The "Yucant" bug is contagious and is spread by notorious spreaders of negativity. They'll find every reason in the world why "you can't" get in shape, "you can't" eat supportively, "you can't" find the time to exercise. Here's a simple suggestion. Look at them. Then look at the Champions who wrote this book. Which group would you rather emulate? The best way to prevent being infected by the "Yucant" bug is to employ yet another simple exercise. Put your hands over your ears and scream as loudly as you possibly can!

This book is going to start with a program, a simple program that you can follow for a week, a month, or literally for the rest of your life, but the book is NOT a program-driven book. The book is an idea-driven book. It's going to plant vital knowledge, treasure, in your head, and that knowledge will not come from me, but from more than 50 Champions of fitness. If you limit your expectations to the hope for a more attractive physique, a better beach body, you're missing out on the true juice of this book. It goes way beyond the ability to control the way you look. It's about empowerment, physical empowerment that can roll over into every aspect of your life.

The Power of Champions is about being a better mother or father, a better spouse, a better friend, a better boss, a better employee, a better leader, a better role model, a better teacher, a better person. You can read at your own pace, but at the very least commit to reading just one page, or better yet, just one short chapter per day. With that slight and gradual injection of new information, the treasure chest reveals itself and the secret is in your hands. Read on. Live like a Champion.

The Traits of Champions

Courage
Heart
Attitude
Muscle
Power
Integrity
Optimism
Nerve

The Program

Components, Rules, and Pitfalls

This is not "your" program in terms of it being a customized program just for you, but this is "a" program that you can begin immediately and adapt as you go. Over time, as you learn from the Champions, you'll be able to modify the program any way you see fit. There are, however, some essential considerations that should remain with you as you refine and develop your own lifetime fitness regimen. There are three components that must be in place, there are five vital rules that must be observed, and there are eight crippling pitfalls you'll want to be aware of to make certain you avoid them.

The Three Essential Components

As with every program I develop, the essential components necessary for physical change are:

- The Right Nutrition
- Moderate Aerobic Exercise
- A Concern For Muscle (Resistance Exercise)

Any program, if it is going to be effective at improving body composition, is going to incorporate all three synergistic elements.

The Five Rules

With a recognition of the three essential components, you must also have a concern for the five vital rules:

You must get both aerobic and anaerobic exercise components integrated into a results-oriented program.

You must "cycle" your training or shift the focus periodically to prevent the process of adaptation from landing you at a plateau.

You must continue to add a new stimulus for greater challenge to keep results consistent and ongoing, which may be an increase in weight, an increase in repetitions, a decrease in rest time between sets, or a strategic combination of exercises that facilitates muscle fatigue.

You must exercise with consistency, committing to between three and six days of exercise per week.

You must be certain to get adequate rest and recuperation.

The Eight Crippling Pitfalls

When someone fails to see a physical payoff from a commitment to exercise, there is always a mistake, always a flaw in the program itself or in the adherence to the strategy. If you learn to recognize and avoid the eight pitfalls capable of crippling the potential for results, you should become and remain the master of your own body.

Pitfall #1: Consuming too much sugar (or refined carbohydrates) on a fat loss program

Pitfall #2: Failing to provide adequate challenge to the working muscles

Pitfall #3: Neglecting protein intake

Pitfall #4: Failing to eat frequently enough

Pitfall #5: Overtraining

Pitfall #6: Believing daily activity "counts" as exercise

Pitfall #7: Failing to ingest calories sufficient to maintain metabolism and supply fuel for activity

Pitfall #8: Failing to schedule down time

As you read through this book, the Champions will help these components, rules, and pitfalls become clearer, but before I turn it over to the Champions, allow me to share the "Champion's Program" in its simplest form.

*   *   *

You'll start with Phase I (what better place to start?). Although each phase is slated for four weeks, there's no reason if you're new to exercise you couldn't stay with this phase for months and continue to see progress. While there are some rules, there is also plenty of room for flexibility. The most important step for you right now is to get started, so view this as a starting point, one that will evolve differently for every reader of this book, but one that in every case is quite capable of serving as the first step toward your physical best.

Notes Regarding Resistance Exercise (weight training): Recommendations will be made in the language of "sets" and "reps." Weight selection is going to be individualized and there will be some trial and error involved. Try to select weights that will bring you to the point of "momentary muscle failure," the point at which you cannot perform another repetition in strict form, within the designated number of reps. In other words, if it specifies "1 set of 8-12 reps," that would indicate that you'd begin a movement attempting to select a weight that allows you to perform at least 8 but not more than 12 repetitions in strict form. Because the recommendation was "1 set," you'd have completed that exercise and would move on to the next. If it specifies "2 sets," after approximately a 90-second rest period, you'd repeat the exercise again.

Notes Regarding Aerobic Exercise: To approximate your Target Heart Zone (THZ), subtract your age from the number 220. That will estimate your Age-Related Maximum Heart Rate. Maximum Heart Rate (MHR) indicates the maximum number of times your heart is capable of beating in a minute. As we age, our maximum heart capacity gradually decreases which is why there is an age-related component to the equation. You do NOT want to exercise at your MHR. THZ is based upon a percentage of MHR and represents a range that would be considered ideal as a gauge to measure aerobic intensity to ensure that aerobic exercise stimulates a training effect. While different agencies may use variations of the formula, for our purposes THZ will be calculated as follows:

Estimating Age-Related Target Heart Zone

$(220 - \text{age}) \times 65\%$ low end of THZ in beats per minute (bpm)

$(220 - \text{age}) \times 85\%$ high end of THZ in beats per minutes

If we were calculating the formula for a 40 year old, it would lay out as follows:

$220 - \text{age} (40) = 180$ (MHR)

$180 \times 65\% = 117$ bpm

$180 \times 85\% = 153$ bpm

THZ = 117 bpm – 153 bpm

Phase I – Muscle Development (4 weeks)

Beginning Exercisers – 1 set of 15 repetitions of each exercise

Intermediate Exercisers – a warm up set of each movement followed by a set where you reach momentary muscle failure at 8-12 reps

Advanced Exercisers – a warm up set of each movement followed by a set where you reach momentary muscle failure at 8-12 reps, and then an increase in weight for another set that brings you to momentary muscle failure between 4 and 6 reps

The Routine

Days: Monday, Wednesday, Friday

The Exercises

- Squat
- Stiff Legged Deadlift
- Bent Over Row
- Chest Press
- Shoulder Press
- Biceps Curl
- Dips
- Calf Raise

Days: Tuesday, Thursday, Saturday

- 90 Abdominal Crunches in sets
  (do as many as you can, rest until you feel ready to complete another set, and continue in this fashion until you reach 90)

- Aerobic Movement: 20 minutes in your THZ

- Aerobic Cool Down

Phase II – Balance and Coordination (4 weeks)

Beginning Exercisers – 1 set of 15 repetitions of each exercise

Intermediate Exercisers – a warm up set of each movement followed by a set where you reach momentary muscle failure at 8-12 reps

Advanced Exercisers – a warm up set of each movement followed by a set where you reach momentary muscle failure at 8-12 reps, and then an increase in weight for another set that brings you to momentary muscle failure between 4 and 6 reps

The Routine

Days: Monday, Wednesday, Friday

The Exercises

- Squat with stability ball
- One Arm Row on stability ball
- Pushups with feet on stability ball
- Shoulder Press seated on stability ball
- Lying Leg Curl with stability ball
- Hip Raise with stability ball

Days: Tuesday, Thursday, Saturday

- 60 Abdominal Crunches on stability ball

- Aerobic Movement 20 minutes staggering high and low ends of the THZ

- Aerobic Cool Down

Phase III – Fat Burning

In this phase, the resistance exercise is performed in a "superset" fashion. Note that the resistance exercises are listed in pairs of exercises (i.e., Lunges superset with Squats). The paired exercises should be performed with little or no rest in between. In other words, in the example noted, immediately upon reaching a point of momentary muscle failure with lunges, you'd begin your squats.

Beginning Exercisers – 1 superset of 15 repetitions per exercise for each pair of movements

Intermediate Exercisers – 2 supersets of 15 repetitions per exercise for each pair of movements

Advanced Exercisers – 3 supersets of 8-15 repetitions per exercise for each pair of movements, increasing the weight slightly on each of the exercises for each consecutive superset

The Routine

Days: Monday, Wednesday, Friday

The Exercises

- Lunge superset with Squat
- One Arm Row superset with Bent Over Lateral Raise
- Side Lateral Raise superset with Shoulder Press
- Dumbbell Fly superset with Chest Press
- Stiff Legged Deadlift superset with Biceps Curl

- Follow weight training with Aerobic Movement for 12 minutes in THZ

- Aerobic Cool Down

Days: Tuesday, Thursday, Saturday

- 30 – 40 minutes of Aerobic Movement at 80% THZ

- 30 – 60 Abdominal Crunches on stability ball

- Advanced exercisers include 2 sets of Hanging Leg Raises or Hip Lifts

Phase I - Muscle Development

Squat

- Head up, back straight, feet pointed slightly out, bend from knees until thighs are parallel with the ground. Allow the hips to flex as you squat, careful to maintain the natural arch of the low back. Do not allow knees past toes. Adjust arm position for balance or, if you're comfortable with the movement, hold a dumbbell in each hand for added resistance. Keep abdominals tight and maintain weight on heels.

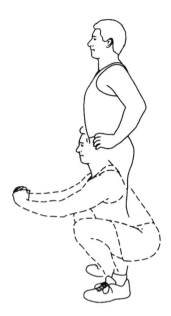

Stiff Legged Deadlift

- Knees slightly bent, head and neck in line with spine. As you bring the upper body forward bending from the hip joint, be certain to maintain the natural arch in the low back.

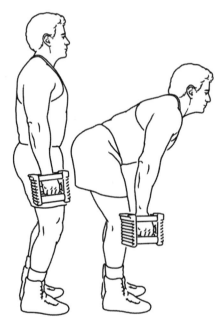

Bent Over Row

- Lift weight to side of chest, keeping elbow close to body. Do all reps to one side. Repeat on other side.

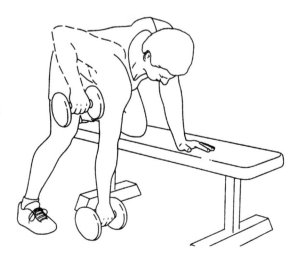

Chest Press

- Upper arms parallel to floor, elbows at 90 degree angle, press to straight arms.

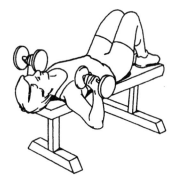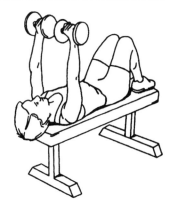

Shoulder Press

- Knees slightly bent, palms in, press to straight arms, rotating to palms forward at end of movement.

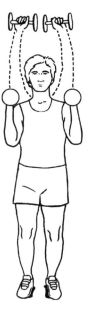

Biceps Curl

- Knees slightly bent, hold weights at sides, palms in. Curl arms toward shoulders, rotating to palms up while beginning curl.

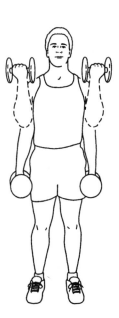

Dips

- Begin with hands supported on bench, arms straight, feet on floor. Bending from the elbows, keeping the elbows close to sides, lower the body downward toward the floor. Then, using the strength of the triceps, press downward as if you're trying to press the bench into the ground, raising your body back to the starting position.

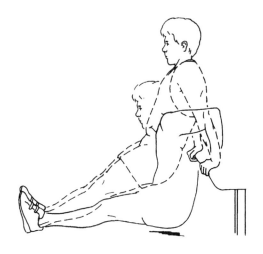

Alternative Dips

- With upper arms parallel to floor, press upward until arms are almost straight with slight bend in the elbows.

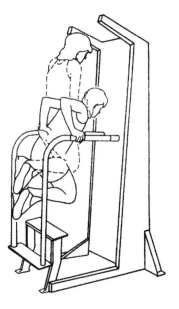

Calf Raise

- Toes on bench or step, knees slightly bent, rise up on toes as high as possible.

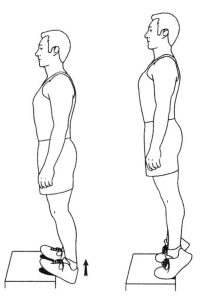

Abdominal Crunches

- Arms crossed, tighten abdominals, raise shoulders and upper back toward ceiling. Keep head and neck in line with spine. Keep low and middle back on floor.

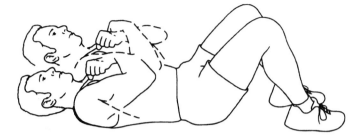

Alternative Abdominal Crunches

- Arms behind head, tighten abdominals, raise shoulders and upper back toward ceiling. Keep head and neck in line with spine. Keep low and middle back on floor.

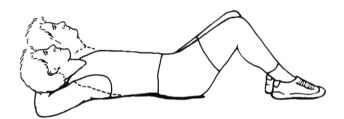

Phase II - Balance and Coordination

Squat with stability ball

- Back straight, bend knees to 90 degree angle. Do not allow knees past toes.

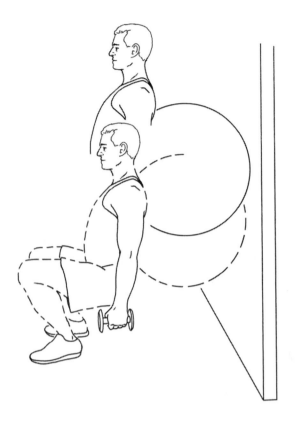

One Arm Row on stability ball

- With feet staggered, arm supported on ball, pull weight to side of chest, keeping elbow close. Keep back straight. Do all reps to one side. Repeat on other side.

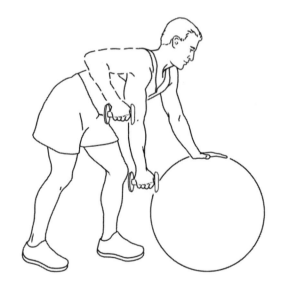

Pushups with feet on stability ball

- Walk out on ball until instep is resting on ball. Lower toward floor keeping head up, back straight, head and neck in line with spine.

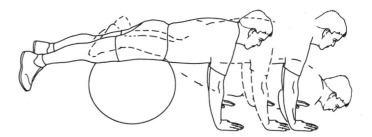

Shoulder Press on stability ball

- Back straight, press dumbbells over head.

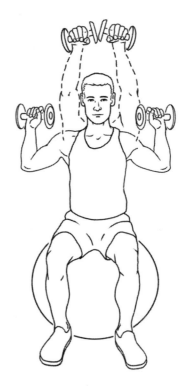

Lying Leg Curl with stability ball

- Feet on ball, roll ball toward body keeping shoulders and upper back on floor with middle and low back straight.

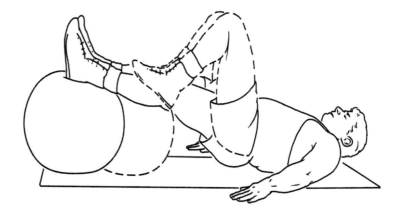

Hip Raise on stability ball

- With legs over ball and back in a neutral position, tighten abdominals and lift hips and low back off the floor.

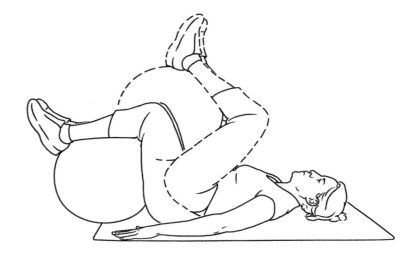

Abdominal Crunch on stability ball

- Support low back on stability ball. Tighten abdominals and bring ribs toward pelvis until shoulders come off the ball.

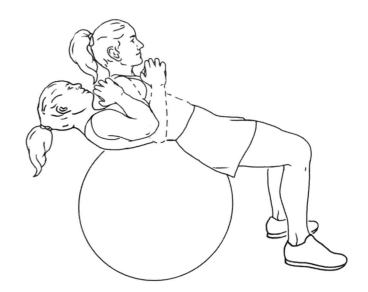

Phase III - Fat Burning

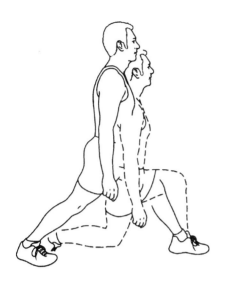

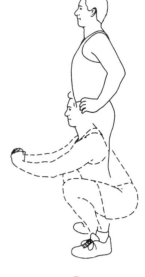

Lunge

Squat

Lunge - In wide stride, legs shoulder width apart, head up, back straight, bend both legs simultaneously until forward thigh is parallel to floor. Do all reps to one side. Repeat on other side.

Squat - Head up, back straight, feet pointed slightly out, bend from knees until thighs are parallel with the ground. Allow the hips to flex as you squat, careful to maintain the natural arch of the low back. Do not allow knees past toes. Adjust arm position for balance or, if you're comfortable with the movement, hold a dumbbell in each hand for added resistance. Keep abdominals tight and maintain weight on heels.

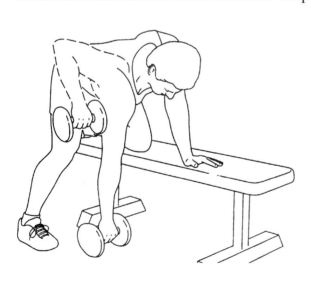

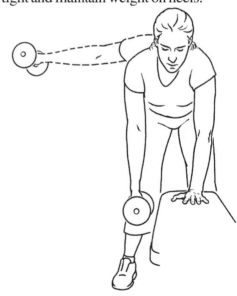

One Arm Row

Bent Over Lateral Raise

One Arm Row - Lift weight to side of chest, keeping elbow close to body. Do all reps to one side. Repeat on other side.

Bent Over Lateral Raise - Knees slightly bent, arm supported, raise arm out to side until parallel with floor. Keep back straight. Do all reps to one side. Repeat on other side.

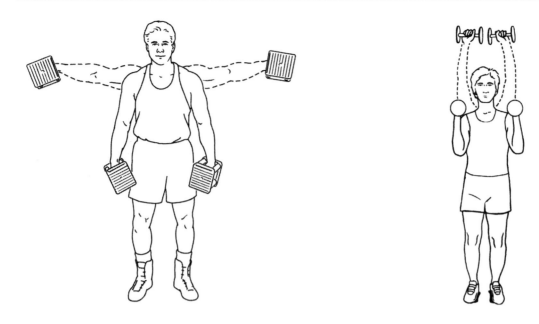

Side Lateral Raise   **Shoulder Press**

Side Lateral Raise - Knees slightly bent, feet shoulder width apart, arms at side with palms in. Lift arms out to side until shoulder height.

Shoulder Press - Knees slightly bent, palms in, press to straight arms, rotating palms forward at end of movement.

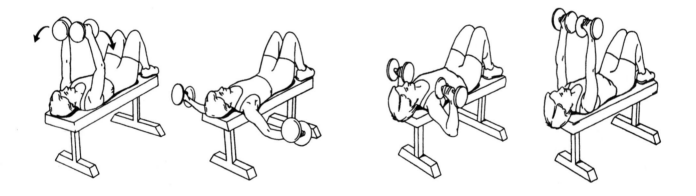

Dumbbell Fly   **Chest Press**

Dumbbell Fly - Lower arms until parallel with floor, elbows slightly bent, palms up.

Chest Press - Upper arms parallel to floor, elbows at 90 degree angle, press to straight arms.

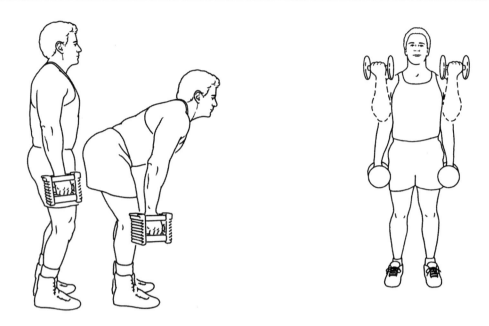

Stiff Legged Deadlift   **Biceps Curl**

Stiff Legged Deadlift - Knees slightly bent, head and neck in line with spine. As you bring the upper body forward bending from the hip joint, be certain to maintain the natural arch in the low back.

Biceps Curl - Knees slightly bent, hold weights at sides, palms in. Curl arms toward shoulders, rotating to palms up while beginning curl.

Abdominal Crunch on stability ball - Support low back on stability ball. Tighten abdominals and bring ribs toward pelvis until shoulders come off the ball.

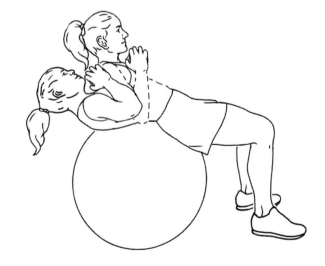

Illustrations provided by Visual Health Information Stretching Charts, Inc., which are the copyrighted property of VHI Inc., P.O. Box 44646, Tacoma, WA 98444, telephone 800-356-0709/253-536-4922.

Introduction to Supportive Nutrition

You already know that Supportive Eating is one of the three essential components. You also have read countless articles and books all serving to confuse the nutritional issue. You've read that sugars are bad, but then you read that chocolate is good. You read that alcohol is bad, but then you read that wine is good. You've read terrible things about the impact of bread on obesity in America, and then you read how a company sponsored study "proved" white bread is . . . well . . . Wonderful. Baffled? Of course you are. It's beyond baffling!

For now I'll make this simple. I'll address three issues that can help you shape your nutrition program.

Calories are Good

Yes, despite what many diet programs would like you to believe, calories are good. Well, at least "good calories in the ideal amounts" would be good. Here's what you should know about calories. They are your fuel. A calorie is not a measure of food as much as it's a unit of heat, and a body with an efficient metabolism is cranking out enough heat to be categorized as a human furnace. Aside from having to maintain a body temperature around 98.6 degrees, every time you contract muscle, every time you think, every time your heart beats, and every time you take a breath calories are burned. Avoid calories and protective processes kick in to slow metabolism to ensure that your body can survive and maintain on fewer calories. That is the complete opposite of what somebody seeking optimal nutrition and improvements in body composition would opt for. You want to get your body good at burning through food. You want to throw fuel in the furnace. You want to eat frequently. The key is when you eat you want to eat metabolically valuable meals.

Eat Often

For the sake of simplicity, you're going to try to get to a meal every 3 – 4 hours, which would amount to between 4 and 6 meals per day. The two potential villains that can contribute to fat accumulation or interrupt the process of fat release are "the unsupportive fats" and "the unsupportive carbs." The unsupportive fats would be hydrogenated fat and, to a lesser degree, saturated fats. Both will be explained in future chapters. The unsupportive carbs would be simple sugars and bleached, processed, and refined grains and flours. They too will be explained in the pages of this book. For now the simple rule is try to eat frequently, ideally every 3-4 hours, and minimize or eliminate intake of the unsupportive fats and the unsupportive carbs.

Lean Protein, Starchy Carb, Fibrous Carb

Now we're left with the question, "What should I eat?" In every one of my books and programs I share the concept of supportive eating, and regardless of the specific goal, if physical improvement is a part of the process, supportive eating is going to require a healthful mix of proteins, complex carbs from natural unrefined sources, fiber, and essential fats. With that in mind I suggest you make the most natural food choices possible (natural food choices are not usually available at a little window you pull up to in your car) and include a lean protein, a starchy carbohydrate, and a fibrous carbohydrate in every meal.

> **Lean proteins** would include chicken breast, turkey breast, egg whites, fish filets, shellfish, soy and tofu, fat-free dairy products, and lean cuts of red meat.

Starchy carbohydrates would include potato, sweet potato, brown rice, whole grains, oatmeal, tomato, peas, and corn.

Fibrous carbs would include broccoli, cauliflower, spinach, mushrooms, peppers, onions, celery, green beans, cabbage, cucumber, and asparagus. Fruits would also be fibrous carbs and, while there is room to include them in meals, they should not make up the mainstay of your diet if fat loss is a goal as the sugar content can interfere with fat release.

These are by no means complete lists but they should offer a starting point. Meals should contain a mix of one food from each group. For example:

- Chicken breast, spinach, sweet potato
- Egg white omelet with green peppers and a side of oatmeal
- Fat-free plain yogurt, blueberries, whole grain cereal

For those times a supportive meal is not accessible or convenient, you should consider the use of a low-sugar or sugar-free meal replacement formula. There are limitless options in the health food stores.

The Mind

Far and away, the most important element in taking charge of your overall health, performance, and physical well being begins within the boundaries of an entity that is all powerful but difficult to define. The Mind. Earl Nightingale in his inspirational wisdom told us "we become what we think about," and whether there is a metaphysical component to this or it is purely motivational, the mind is the driving force. You have the desire; hopefully at this point you believe in the possibility of a rewarding physical payoff. Now it's up to you to grab hold, to master your mindset to one that goes beyond possibility into the realm of commitment. The two-part commitment is simple. Wait, before I share it, let's do a test.

Stand Up!

Did you do it this time? If you did, get ready, your life's about to move in an incredible new direction. If you didn't, well . . . I can only do so much. I can give you the information, but it's up to you to use it and to incorporate another vital element. The follow-through. Make up your mind. You can do this. You WILL do this.

With some preliminary direction, here is the two part commitment:

- Read at least one page, or ideally one short chapter, per day
- Make your exercise and supportive eating a priority and keep your commitment to follow through

Simple enough, right? OK, get ready for your knowledge base to expand as I turn you over to the scores of true professionals making significant differences in people's lives. The rest of the book is written by those I've aptly named, "The Champions!" Every once in awhile I may interject, but I am but one voice among many. You've already started amassing a virtual wealth of knowledge compiled by some of the most outstanding minds to have ever entered the fitness field.

We're going to begin by allowing the Champions to share some stories and some inspirational words that can help you understand the essence of the journey. Fitness is not a goal to be tackled instantaneously. It's the result of figuratively putting one foot in front of the other. Initially a step requires thought and concentration, but with time and stick-to-it-iveness, the steps become automatic and the results become thrilling.

Commit, now, to read just a little bit each day and the steps to your ultimate achievement begin to stack upon themselves until it's hard to believe this ever required what at this moment may feel like effort. You've got momentum. Don't stop here . . . turn the page and begin walking along the path to Excellence.

Phil Kaplan, ACE, NSCA

President
Phil Kaplan's Fitness Associates
1304 SW 160th Avenue, #337
Sunrise, FL 33326
561-204-2014
www.philkaplan.com

SECTION ONE
The Attitude of Champions

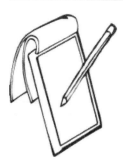

Notes from Phil

If I tried to accurately define "attitude," I'd be venturing into a complex land of psychological principles where those who commit their lives to the study of human behavior congregate, debate, argue, and re-define. I won't go there. I'll make it simple. Your attitude is in great part a choice. Champions choose to enter a state of readiness, a willingness to move forward and respond to any situation that may arise along the way.

I recently overheard two teenage girls walking out of a sub shop, verbally tearing apart the girl working behind the counter. "Did you see the way she looked at you? She needs a 'tude adjustment."

'Tude can be destructive, 'tude can be repulsive, or . . . given the right outlook, consciously choosing an empowering 'tude can be the equivalent of electing to use rocket fuel to power the journey to your dreams. Champions rarely get caught up in the traps sprung from a bad-itude run rampant. As Champion Jonathan Ross will share in this section, the right attitude combined with tiny steps in a consistent direction create a formula for astounding achievement. Champion Brian J. Johnston follows with his assertion that consistency is something that can be cultivated, and while he'll emphasize that the outcome you seek may not be "quick and easy," he'll lay out a formula that allows you to master an attitude founded in consistency.

Champion Tony Rodriguez, no stranger to the concept of "coaching," will teach you that your best coach lies within, and with SMART goal setting, your 'tude catches fire! Champion Linda Cook then shares some insight into an element desired by Champions and novices alike . . . POWER!

Champion Charmas B. Lee wraps the section up with seven principles that have allowed even those with significant challenges to excel!

Get ready . . . it's 'tude adjusting time!

Excellence – A Culmination of Tiny Steps by Jonathan Ross

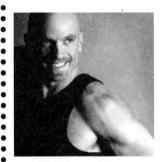

Champion Jonathan Ross of Bowie, Maryland is dedicated to making you fit in the body, ready in the mind, and high in spirit. He believes that happiness is when what you say, what you think, and what you do are in harmony.

What's the most important change you can make to achieve your fitness goals?

Even with an abundance of fitness information, millions of decent people are continually frustrated in their efforts at physical improvement. Our society's approach and attitudes about fitness doom many sincere efforts at physical change to failure. Rather than integrate exercise into our lives, we add it as another item on our already overcrowded "to-do" lists. In making our lives more efficient, we compartmentalize everything – including efforts at fitness. What can you do to overcome this?

To see massive results, you continuously make small changes and integrate them into your lifestyle. I'll help you identify the most important changes to make. You'll learn about my once obese mother's journey to fitness and health. She has made amazing progress by approaching change in the manner I share here. Her journey was much more daunting than what many of you may ever face.

We pride ourselves on productivity. In keeping a busy schedule, we separate our responsibilities. We have work time, family time, play time, personal time, *fitness* time, and we keep them all isolated from one another. Consider the person who commits to an hour of exercise daily. They drive to the gym and circle the parking lot to get a spot close to the building so they don't have a long walk to the treadmill. At work, they take the elevator instead of the stairs and have some doughnuts thinking, "Why not? I worked out this morning." Their *fitness hour* is the only time physical activity enters their day. What's happening during the other 23 hours? While it may appear that this person is making an effort to achieve their goals, separating fitness from the rest of their life leads to a disconnection, ultimately manifesting itself in frustration with lack of results and discouragement. For permanent results to become reality, the changes we make must become integrated into our daily routines.

This is a world where instant coffee isn't fast enough. Incessant sales pitches for products that promise massive results effortlessly make it increasingly difficult to accept that fitness success takes more than pills and a few days of dieting. Our eternally busy culture has conditioned us to demand what we want when we want it. The result: Good people with good intentions spending good money on fast fitness frauds. Often, the number of changes you must make feels overwhelming. You may have felt that if you can't make all the changes you need to at once, then you shouldn't bother because you'll just be wasting your time and effort. It doesn't have to be that way. A single change can begin your fitness journey. It did for my mother.

I had two parents, but I had more parents than most people. In fact, I had 800 pounds of parents. My father was 424 pounds, my mother 370. My father died several years ago at the relatively young age of 56. This was a critical turning point for my mother and me. My father's death from his poor lifestyle choices was the flashpoint for my career as a personal trainer with a mission to help you reach your physical potential. For my mother, Patricia, it was a massive wake up call. She faced her own mortality.

My mother's results are directly related to integration of fitness into her life. Gradual changes made all the difference to the end result. The first change was to her eating habits. By consuming adequate amounts of healthier foods, she lost 90 pounds. Each small nutrition change played a role in delivering this result. If she had tried to make them all at once, it would have been too overwhelming for her. Another client of mine went from drinking a six-pack of soda daily to none and lost 20 pounds from this one change.

My mother had lost significant weight, but she was compartmentalizing by limiting her changes to nutrition. She struggled to continue her progress. Frustrated that she had reached a plateau, she finally realized that it was time to get moving – literally. Again, she began with small changes. She took swimming classes at a local college. She took group exercise classes. She met with me twice weekly for resistance training. By gradually integrating what I was teaching her about exercise into her life, her weight loss resumed. However, this time was different.

She integrated fitness with her social time, play time, and family time; her life became infused with fitness. Fitness was no longer a separate, unattainable goal. She not only lost more weight, but felt physically more confident and capable. She wasn't just losing weight; she was getting leaner – losing body fat and adding muscle. She lived the connection between nutrition and activity. She lost another 80 pounds, for a total of 170. She looked and felt dramatically better. She would occasionally miss a workout, but refused to let temporary disruptions become permanent obstructions. She never quit and is always improving, always progressing. Her old lifestyle is several years and 170 pounds ago. She lives a vibrant life in a body she loves. Just look at the difference each small step made for her!

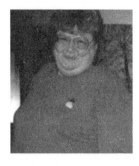

Pat Ross - 1995

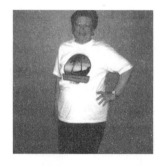

Pat Ross - 2002

You may have struggled for decades with your weight. Imagine...if you had ignored the fads and built upon small, reasonable changes, you would already have achieved your fitness goals by now. This illustrates the folly and frustration of following the fads. If you've chased the latest 30-day fitness craze, followed every fad diet, and told yourself repeatedly that you'll start over and do better next week, you may have lost the same 20 pounds over and over again. Many clients have shared with me the various amounts of weight that they have lost by dieting. Often the total of weight is close to what they currently weigh! They tell me the diets "worked." However, they're still asking for help. If you're losing the same weight repeatedly, dieting is not working. The frustration of continuous effort without consistent results has likely dealt a crushing blow to your belief that change is possible, yet you still desire change. Desire without belief that change is possible drives the marketing for bogus products. There's little risk if it doesn't work. After all, there's always the next diet.

Let's discuss dieting. The word "diet" literally means "manner of living" – a permanent lifestyle, not a short-term radical change to achieve a goal weight on a goal date. It's integration, not isolation. It's a way of life. How ironic – a word intended to describe our way of life now represents an extreme example of compartmentalizing fitness. The current use of "diet" implies restriction and deprivation. This isn't a way of life that I'm interested in.

It's imperative to make changes gradually. My clients have made massive physical transformations by consistently building on small changes. For healthy changes to take hold, you need to embrace them and weave them into the fabric of your life. It's not easy to change lifestyle habits so don't expect perfection.

Continuous progress is crucial to fitness success. You simply must take a step in the right direction. If you consider all the changes you need to make, they'll seem overwhelming or you'll try to do too much too quickly and give up in frustration. Don't be a perfectionist, be a "progressionist." Consistently improve by building on small changes. Here's how to be a progressionist.

Identify two things to do immediately that will move you in a positive direction. Allow those changes to take hold – to become part of you, to become permanent. At regular intervals – weekly, bi-weekly, monthly – commit to more changes. It can be anything! Replace one soda daily with water. Eat breakfast consistently. Schedule your workouts like other important activities. Try a new fitness class or new healthy recipe weekly. Play tag with the kids. Park in the "fitness section" of the parking lot (far enough away to require a bit of walking). Skip the chips that come with a sandwich. You control what you eat and what you do.

What's the most important change for you? The first one! The beauty is that you decide what that change is. Begin with the changes most significant to you. It worked for my mother and it will work for you. Take action. Every step brings you closer to making your fitness vision a reality. Enjoy your journey, one day your results will just appear.

Jonathan Ross, ACE, NSCA

2003 Personal Fitness Professional Magazine Personal Trainer of the Year Award – Personal Training Director
Aion Fitness – Fitness for a Lifetime...and the Time of Your Life!
301-367-6843
Jonathan.Ross@thepowerofchampions.com

Cultivating Consistency by Brian J. Johnston

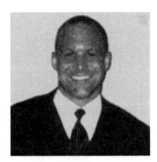

Champion Brian J. Johnston of Atlanta, Georgia has been empowering clients and educating trainers to achieve their fitness purpose for more than a decade. Begin your evolution today.

Question: What do Rome, the Great Pyramids, the Grand Canyon and the Earth have in common with your current physical condition?

Answer: They all required a great deal of time to achieve!

For many, achieving goals is an all-or-nothing proposition. Many who begin a health and fitness program expect to see results overnight. Those who succeed recognize that change and growth of any type require a consistent investment of time and effort.

Before we get into the mechanics of success, please take a moment to consider the following...

Is Success Luck or Choice? You Decide!

Below are three of the most important questions you'll ever answer:

    1. Do you believe there is something you could specifically do in the next 30 days to make your personal, family or business life better?

    2. Do you believe there is something you could specifically do in the next 30 days to make your personal, family or business life worse?

    3. Do you believe every choice you make has an end result?

If you answered "Yes" to all three questions, you subscribe to the following philosophy: I don't care how good or bad my past has been. I don't care how difficult my circumstances may be at this particular moment. There is something I can do right now that can make my future better or worse… and the choice is mine!

Yes, the choice to either forge ahead or fall behind is truly yours! If you commit to learning (and consistently applying) the principles, techniques and strategies in *The Power of Champions*, you can experience a new level of health and fitness satisfaction.

But let me warn you: My fellow Champions and I will not tell you what you want to hear. We're going to tell you what you need to hear, even though it may be difficult to face initially.

Let's get one thing straight: despite the billions of dollars the weight loss and fitness industry generates trying to convince you otherwise, getting from where you currently are to where you ultimately want to be is not "quick and easy." While the offers may sometimes be tempting, you know the road labeled "quick and easy" is not the correct path! Achieving worthwhile goals requires a consistent investment of time and effort on your part.

The alarming rise of obesity and other health concerns is proof positive that believing any single action will ultimately result in success is going to leave you frustrated. The best tool you can acquire for achieving success is an understanding of the overall requirements for physical improvement. Buying self-help books or tapes, attending seminars or therapy, purchasing pills, powders and patches, and ordering the "latest and greatest" weight loss gizmos and gadgets may summon a burst of motivation but, in and of themselves, not one of these actions can offer the answer to America's weighty woes. Even those who dive into long-term health club memberships generally abandon the effort by discontinuing their health club visits while continuing to pay hefty membership fees for several years!

So, what is the answer?

It all begins with consistency. In simple terms, do what you're supposed to do, when you're supposed to do it – consistently!

Consistent effort and dedication is needed to remain faithful to your significant other, achieve a promotion at work, get good grades in school and keep your checkbook balanced. The same applies to your fitness program. It's an immutable law of the universe that you can't get 'something for nothing.' Basically:

The rewards you receive will be in direct proportion to the consistent effort you put forth!

By now you may be thinking that changing an old habit, achieving a healthy goal or maintaining a superior state of mind can be extremely difficult, if not seemingly impossible, at times. And it can be downright maddening to try repeatedly, only to fail repeatedly. Perhaps you have already given up on yourself. But please don't. You can succeed at anything you set your mind to if you're willing to back it up with an unstoppable attitude and consistent effort!

Program with a Purpose – Find Your 'Why'

When you are truly motivated to achieve a goal – if it's something you really desire – a consistent and Herculean effort is usually applied! To maintain momentum and stay the course through the ups and downs, it's imperative to consistently focus on your purpose…or why you ultimately want to achieve the goal.

It's incredibly difficult to remain consistent unless you are motivated by a higher purpose. Generally speaking, nebulous, weak or selfish goals result in failure. Get clear on what it is you really want to accomplish.

Keeping Your Perspective in Perspective

To get from where you currently are to where you ultimately want to be, first determine your starting point, both physically and mentally.

Just as a health assessment precedes the development of a fitness or nutrition program, a mental makeover is equally important to both setting goals and developing the strategies you will use to achieve them. When something is 'real' to you, those thoughts tend to become your daily reality.

We Are What We Believe Ourselves To Be

If you believe you are fat, clumsy, shy, stupid or not good enough, chances are your life will be a self-fulfilling prophecy. Similar to a computer, practically every action you take (or don't take) is based on thoughts (beliefs) that are mentally programmed into your belief system. For more information about positive self-talk, be sure to read 'Mental Conditioning – Self Talk' by Champion Tony Avilez.

So How Can You Reprogram Yourself for Success?

First, realize you are capable of more than you think. Many times the only difference between success and failure are but small things done consistently.

Next, think success! Dismiss all thoughts of possible failure. Eliminate undesirable four-letter words such as "can't," "don't" or "won't" from your vocabulary. Instead, let the command "I will succeed" become your daily mantra!

Follow Through If You Want to Finish Strong

Knowing your starting point and the necessary changes you need to make are important, but it's only part of the picture. You must consistently follow through each day on whatever actions are required to achieve your goals.

Whether it's incorporating additional cardio activities into your week, waking up an hour earlier to workout, or setting aside an evening to prepare your meals for the week, if you consistently apply yourself each day, you can achieve your goals!

Helpful Hints for Staying Consistent

To remain consistent, you must enjoy what you're doing. Here's how:

- Make it fun.
- Vary your routine. Athletes call this cross training. Alternating physical activities throughout your week can help develop different sets of muscles, improve skills and eliminate boredom.
- Keep your brain busy. Make the most of your time by reading on the stationary bike or treadmill, or listening to your favorite music while lifting weights.
- Make activity a social event. Get a workout partner or join a group. This is great for motivation and accountability. Playing outdoor games with your kids counts as exercise too. Take a walk or bike ride with your family, or spend the afternoon together at the park or pool.

Reward Yourself

To reinforce consistent behavior, make yourself a deal. Treat yourself to a new pair of shoes or an outfit once you've completed a full month of consistent physical activity. Take your significant other out for a nice dinner after following your nutrition plan consistently for the month. Put a specified amount of money in a jar every time you workout and use it to buy yourself something special at the end of the year.

Continuous progress requires continuous effort...

Remember, the more consistent you are, the easier it gets. Consistency forces your body to adapt and become more efficient each time.

By incorporating a variety of movements and manipulating the frequency, intensity, duration and volume, you can avoid plateaus, boredom, reduce your risk of injury and enjoy continuous progress.

Becoming stronger, leaner, more radiant, sexy, better at sports, having more energy to play with your kids, fitting into a smaller dress or pair of pants, or even getting a second glance from that someone special are but a few of the physical and mental benefits you can expect from applying yourself - consistently!

By implementing these strategies you will return to your career, family and life with increased confidence, a sense of accomplishment, contagiously enthused, rejuvenated...evolved!

Brian J. Johnston, NCCPT CPT/PT Certification Instructor, ISSA CFT1/SPN

404-451-4170
888-353-5303
Brian.Johnston@thepowerofchampions.com
www.evolve-now.com

Be Your Own "Fitness Coach" by Tony Rodriguez

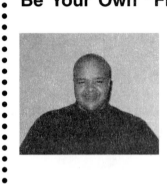

Champion Tony Rodriguez of East Setauket, New York owns a personal training facility that specializes in training the 'baby boomer' client. His experience includes the creation of a national corporate wellness program for Eastman Kodak.

Every year, right after New Year's Day every gym in America is busting at the seams.

Memberships are highest at this time of year. All of the excessive holiday eating is on the minds of every person making the resolution to "finally get fit."

Most people start this journey with the best of intentions. They make up their minds that enough is enough and they jump in with both feet. Enthusiasm is high and a leaner, more toned, fitter body is envisioned for the coming spring and summer seasons. So why does this positive journey toward ultimate personal fitness vanish as quickly as it began? There are many different reasons but my experience training and coaching hundreds of clients over the past 10 years has shown me one common denominator pertaining to this failure to achieve success - the lack of a clear plan of action toward achieving a long-range goal.

Recently I mentioned to one of my clients that my goal for next year was to purchase the new 2005 Ford Mustang. I'm somewhat of a car nut and this car has been on my mind for the last few months. My client, who is a CPA and makes a living helping people set and reach their financial goals, asked me nonchalantly what my plan of action was. He knows how big I am on the process of goal setting and assumed that my plan to purchase my dream car was in place. I didn't have a plan in place. I realized that every year I say I'm finally getting my dream car but never do. Why? No plan! The likelihood of achieving this goal for me was diminished by the fact that I had not set small, attainable goals that would finally lead to getting the car of my dreams.

Many people take on the task of improving their health and fitness levels the same way. It's like taking an automobile road trip to a new destination without a map or gas in the tank. Wouldn't that be foolish? Well, a large majority of us take on a fitness program the same way. The process of goal setting is the same, regardless of the goal. It's a simple but extremely powerful tool that's been used by most high achievers to reach sometimes extraordinary goals.

A few years ago, I accepted the position of head coach for an online fitness coaching company. I assisted the management team in developing a coaching methodology that helped clients achieve their health and fitness goals. What made this methodology unique was the fact that the only interaction we had with these clients was through the company web site or the telephone. We had to empower these clients to take charge of their health and improve their fitness levels without being there in person to offer encouragement and motivation. The one concept that enabled us to do this effectively was the process of goal setting.

Coaching and goal setting are almost synonymous. Realize, though, that coaching is not therapy. It focuses only on the present and the future. Therapy goes deeply into the past, as well as the present and future.

Using my online coaching experience, I began using these techniques with clients at my facility and the results have been fabulous. Allow me to share, in detail, this powerful process with you so that you can begin to enjoy your health and fitness dreams by being your own fitness coach.

There are certain factors that must be present pertaining to successful goal achievement. I found that a long-range goal should be no longer than 3 months ahead. In other words, what can you safely achieve within a 12–week time period? This is especially important when it pertains to weight loss. Many times an unrealistic weight loss goal is set (e.g., 50 pounds in 3 months) and, when that goal is not met, many quit and feel the effort wasn't worth the results achieved. A more realistic goal would be a 12-pound weight loss (1 pound per week) accomplished by small weekly and daily goals that would contribute toward that long-range goal. It's a simple yet strong approach that, if followed through, can help you achieve many of your aspirations.

A strong plan of action toward successful goal achievement needs to adhere to certain criteria. This criterion involves S.M.A.R.T. goals. S.M.A.R.T. is an acronym for *S*pecific, *M*easurable, *A*ttainable, *R*ealistic, and *T*ime-oriented.

Specific - Your goal needs to be stated in great detail and be very specific. For example, instead of saying "I want to lose weight in the next 3 months," you should be very specific with a realistic weight loss number, such as "I want to lose 12 pounds in 3 months." Have a precise plan on how to achieve that weight loss goal.

Once that's done, write down your plan. Ask yourself, "What am I going to do on a weekly and daily basis to achieve this goal?" I found that the clients I coached online achieved greater success when the goals were written down and were as specific as possible. I met with each client once a week and a weekly "fitness contract" would be in place after each session where the goals for the upcoming week would be listed. Examples of items in this contract include:

- I'll exercise in the morning before work at my local gym with my friend, Tom at 7:00 a.m.
- I'll wake up an hour earlier to walk on my treadmill between 6:00 a.m. – 6:30 a.m.
- I'll eat a healthy breakfast each morning until my next online session.

Bottom line - the more specific and detailed you are in stating your goal, the more likely you are to achieve it. I strongly suggest you write down these goals and create a "contract" with yourself on a weekly or even daily basis, whatever is feasible for you. Keep it simple but be consistent.

Measurable - I'm a big believer in establishing both objective and subjective baseline measurements with all of my clients. How much of each of these measurements depends on the client. The point is that you have something that you can look at over time to sustain motivation and show progress. Examples include:

- Monthly measurements of certain body areas, such as chest, waist, thighs, etc.
- Heightened awareness of how certain clothes fit
- Improved energy levels over time
- Weigh-ins – this can be done on a weekly, bi-weekly, or monthly basis

Note - I'm not a big fan of using body weight alone to gauge progress since the emphasis should be on body composition changes (less fat, more muscle). Realistically, however, we all like to see and should expect an eventual lower number on the scale. That lower number makes every client smile. *The Power of Champions* offers two great resources for information on body composition: 'Fat Loss Rather than a Focus on Pounds' by Champion Amy Powlison and 'Measuring and Using Body Composition Effectively' by Champion Lisa Martin.

Pick what works for you. Again, keep it simple but consistent. Establish a schedule for the objective measurements (weekly, monthly, etc.).

Attainable – Establish goals that are important to you and can be achieved in small attainable steps. Many clients train with me two times a week. Knowing the importance of at least two or three additional strength or cardio-related workouts, we agree to small daily goals before we meet again. For example, if we are training together on Monday and Friday, my clients set a daily goal for Wednesday to jog at the local school track for 30 minutes. A small nutritional goal might be to drink 5 glasses of water for the next day and a reduction in coffee from the usual 4 cups per day to only 2 cups. The long-range goal could be 8-10 glasses of water per day and no coffee but, like they say, we need to crawl before we walk and walk before we run. Small attainable goals are the way to go. Success begets success and the achievement of these small goals helps establish this fact.

Realistic - Realistic goals that can be achieved in a certain time period ensure success. Often clients want to achieve an unrealistic goal such as a "bikini body " in 12 weeks. I ask each client that starts our weight-management program the same question to help ascertain a realistic weight loss goal. What was their lowest body weight in the past 10 years? If a person currently weighs 200 pounds and strives to be 185 pounds and has been that weight in the last 10 years, that would be a very realistic goal to achieve in the next 12 weeks. If their weight in the last 10 years was dramatically lower (165 lbs.), I'd explain to them what can safely be achieved in 3 months and that it may take an additional 6-12 weeks after the initial 3 months to achieve their eventual weight-loss goal.

Time-oriented - Committing to a specific timeframe increases successful goal achievement. Commit to achieving a specific goal by a certain time and do your best to achieve it in that timeframe. If that time period ends without achieving that goal, don't beat yourself up. Step back and take an honest look at what happened, then set up another plan to achieve that goal in a safe but specific time period.

Using established coaching skills, including goal setting strategies, toward achieving your optimum health and fitness could be a rewarding experience. It all begins with that first step in the right direction. Take that step today!

Tony Rodriguez, CPFT, MES

Studio One Fitness & Nutrition
196 Belle Mead Road, Suite 5
East Setauket, NY 11733
631-941-2746
Tony.Rodriguez@thepowerofchampions.com

Power! by Linda Cook

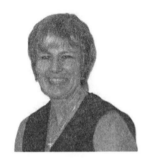

Champion Linda Cook of Springboro, Ohio is a 55-year old grandmother with a passion for helping people gain control of their health and body. Teaching them to stay pain-free through exercise, she gives them the power to gain self-esteem they never had, or thought they'd lost.

My husband and I were watching Gene Roddenberry's *Andromeda* last night. Pretty powerful show. After all, this leader and his team are trying to save not only our little world, but the entire universe as well!

…then the power went out. No, not just the power oozing from every pore of Kevin Sorbo's body (for those of you who don't know, he's the captain of the Andromeda), but the electrical power to our house. All we could do was sit there in the dark; maybe find our flashlights, candles, or anything to keep us from stumbling around blindly.

What if it was gone forever?

What if a giant negative force suddenly zapped our entire world's energy?

What if the power never came back?

It's obvious this morning the power did come back "on." After all, I'm sitting here pounding away at my keyboard again. What created the problem? More than likely, somewhere along the line, there was a break in the power conduit. It had no way to get from its source to our house. Somewhere, someone had to make the connection again. That's what we're here to do for you!

Where did all the power go?

Let's consider even the remote possibilities for our power outage. Somehow, we all know that the power plant, our car, or even our bodies can't function without fuel. No Fuel = No Power! If our tank is empty, we stop. If we try to put diesel, water, oil, or any other fuel in when gasoline is required, we still can't move. Not only do engines require enough fuel to create power; they require the right mix of fuels. Our team of Champions is devoted to helping you determine which fuels create your best mix. Their advice will also be your guidebook for how often you need to refuel, and how much.

So where's the fire?

Now we're pumping in the right fuel to produce energy. We're doing it on a regular basis. But the engine still won't turn over! The lights aren't on. Maybe there's no spark to ignite the fuel? My bet is that's why you're reading this book. You need the initial spark to light your fire. We're here to kindle your desire and make change possible.

Okay—let's move!

Engines started; the spark worked! But still no power to turn the wheels! Maybe we have a breakdown in the delivery system, or not enough oxygen getting to the flame. That part has to come from you. Here's where you have to use movement to build and strengthen your pumps and to provide the pipeline for getting power delivered when and where it's needed. This delivery system must be in constant motion to keep power consistent. Otherwise, your power will periodically die on you and have to be restarted. Any good mechanic will tell you: stop-and-go driving is extremely hard on engines!

Again, our team of Champions provides you with the tools to define how often, how hard, and how long— the frequency, intensity, and duration for your motion. For "what" to do, we've given you a roadmap, but the details are up to you. Make your routine something you enjoy—with some variety thrown in to keep it working for you. Even a beautiful drive gets dull if you take it every day.

But what does it all mean?

Now that we've got the *Power*, what are we going to do with it? What does it mean to us? Since I don't believe that one source can have <u>all</u> the answers, I asked some of my closest friends, including some co-workers and clients, what power means to them. Here are some of their answers:

- Strength
- Choice
- Speed
- Freedom
- Stamina
- Spirit
- Opportunity
- Leadership
- Being able to live life passionately
- Holding on to a dream
- Living life one moment at a time
- The ability to do something above and beyond

Whew…quite a list! But I have one more to add…

At the beginning of her training session a few weeks ago, I asked one of my most powerful clients to give me her definition. I told her not to answer me then, but to really think about it. At the end of our session, she said: "Answering your question is easy… Control!"

I laughed,"You're not helping me much! That's my definition."

"I think I can, I think I can, I know I can….."

First, start with the right fuel—for us humans, that's food. Remember: No Fuel = No Power. It must be the right fuel for the job, in the right amounts, at the right time. Some will give you almost instant energy, some will be used to help you think, some will be used to repair tissue, and some will be stored in muscle fiber or as fat cells for later use. You'll find your best mix, guided by the advice of our Champions in Section Six, 'Eat Like a Champion.'

Second, start moving. No Motion = No Power! But don't "just do it"…learn how to do it right. Very few of us are superhuman with an innate ability to change just moving to functional motion. To find a trainer near you go to www.thepowerofchampions.com. Allow yourself full and free use of your physical ability. This will give you the self-confidence required to make things happen.

Third, keep on fueling and moving. Consistency is over half the battle. There is no instant, everlasting, one-time *Power* pill. With appropriate motion and nutrition, your strength, speed and stamina will be under your control. Your energy source will be protected against breakdown or blow-up. When decisions need to be made, and action taken, you won't have to wait for someone else. You will have the freedom to choose. Champion Brian J. Johnston's chapter, 'Cultivating Consistency,' provides guidelines and tips for getting and staying consistent.

Keep it burning!

We have lights now, but sometimes they flicker or fade; sometimes they almost go totally out, if only for a second. What have we missed? We've confirmed that we have enough fuel, and the right mix of fuels pumped in at the right time. We've started that fuel burning with a spark, and kept it hot by fanning it with movement, making the mix perfect for power when and where it's needed. But what if our needs change?

Recognize that what we're trying to do, and the body we're trying to do it with, is always changing. We want it to! Sometimes we're asking for more, or maybe just something different. *Power* demands to run a race, overcome an illness, think through a problem, or work marathon hours are totally different. It's really okay to change your preferred habits for something special. This is not regression, but the ability to adapt. You need to supply power and delivery methods matched to your life at the moment. Reach inside yourself, your mind, body, and spirit; use the Champions as your guides, and take the challenge to go above and beyond!

There you have it! The lights are staying on. We've given you our secret formula. You now have the power and control to save the universe - or maybe just yourself to begin with.

But wait! There's something that perhaps you didn't count on. Having this *Power* means that you also have to assume responsibility for it. You have to make your own decisions, do what has to be done, and that includes sharing your knowledge with others. Now you know why we're here...

What you do next with your *Power* is up to you...

Where do you want it to take you next week; next year; for the rest of your life?

Fulfill your desire....use your *Power* to become a Champion!

Linda Cook, ACE CES/LWMC/GFI

Your Personal Best!
20 Southridge Court
Springboro, OH 45066
937-748-7363
Linda.Cook@thepowerofchampions.com
www.ictraining.com/YourPersonalBest!

Achieving Success: The Step-Wise Approach by Charmas B. Lee

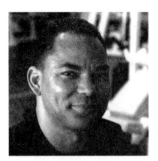

Champion Charmas B. Lee of Colorado Springs, Colorado provides services for private and corporate fitness, physician- and physical-therapy referred clients, and sport-specific enhancement. He is Fitness Trainer at the USAF Academy Preparatory School, founder of Speed T & F and owner of Building Better Bodies.

Several years ago I had the opportunity to work with a young man I'll call John in a program based out of Colorado Springs called Speed Inc.

Although he was only 14 or 15 years old at the time, his biological age did not match his chronological age. John stood almost 6 feet tall and weighed about 140 pounds. John had a severe learning disability, an issue he has since overcome. He will not only graduate from Penn State University this year, but he has also qualified for the 2004 Olympic Trials.

The diabetic, the work-at-home mom, or the senior citizen who is delaying the onset of osteoporosis through strength training could easily achieve John's success. I have chosen his story because it reinforces how we all have the innate ability to improve our current level of fitness and go to the next level. Here are the training principles that you can implement to achieve your personal success and beat the odds!

- **Training Principle 1:** Find out what works, then do it!

- **Training Principle 2:** Implement a plan with simple goals

- **Training Principle 3:** Consistency - stay the course

- **Training Principle 4:** Capture the vision

- **Training Principle 5:** Eat like a Champion

- **Training Principle 6:** Don't ignore red flags

- **Training Principle 7:** Team approach

Here are the details!

Training Principle 1: Find out what works, then do it! Plan activities that you enjoy and will look forward to performing often. Whatever activities you choose should stimulate both your mind and body. It is very difficult to maintain mental fortitude if you dread your workouts.

Make sure your training program complements your goals and personality. Consider inviting a friend to workout with you – preferably someone at the same fitness level or a little higher. Or do you prefer to workout alone? Do you prefer to workout at home or at a health club? Not sure. Read Champion Joe Stankowski's chapter, 'Is a Health Club Right for Me?' While both cardio and strength are important to any fitness program, depending on your fitness goals, determine which one you should emphasize.

Training Principle 2: Implement a plan with simple goals. Goal setting should be specific, measurable and attainable. Write your goals down using positive language. When developing a plan, you want to keep your long-term goals in sight but develop a plan that includes short-term goals along the way. Champion Tony Rodriguez shares goal setting techniques that have helped his clients achieve success in his chapter, 'Be Your Own "Fitness Coach".'

You have heard it a thousand times – those who fail to plan, plan to fail. A good plan requires preparation, should be purposeful, provide direction and be time efficient. Champion Doug Jackson offers great tips for getting the most out of your workouts in a short amount of time in his chapter, 'Time Efficient Workouts.'

Intrinsic rewards are just as important as extrinsic rewards. Intrinsic rewards include improved energy, self-confidence, lower blood pressure and a stronger, more efficient heart. Extrinsic rewards are great motivational tools as you reach your short-term goals. For example, treat yourself to a massage when you complete your first 5K. This can be a very motivating goal.

You never know how far getting started can take you!

Training Principle 3: Consistency - stay the course. Make no excuses! Reasons are why we succeed, excuses are why we fail. The best-laid plans often fall by the wayside when the hard work begins. Schedule your workouts a month ahead of time in your planner and stick to it as you would any other important appointment. If something unavoidable does comes up and you cannot perform the entire workout, decide what you can do. For example, I keep a jump rope in my car. If I am under a time constraint and can't perform 40 minutes of cardio, I will jump rope for 12-18 minutes at a higher intensity instead.

Champion Brian J. Johnston's chapter, 'Cultivating Consistency,' can help you reach the next level.

Training Principle 4: Capture the vision. Develop a clarifying statement that defines what you are trying to achieve. This will help you stick to your purpose, provide you with a sense of ownership and keep you motivated. For example: My purpose for training is to prevent chronic disease in my life.

Training Principle 5: Eat like a Champion. Placing predisposed genetics aside, nutrition can account for at least 50% of your production. Fuel your body properly so you can call upon energy at any given moment. To learn more about how to efficiently and supportively fuel your body, read Champion Jason Robertson's chapter, 'The Right Nutrition.'

Training Principle 6: Don't ignore red flags. Listen to your body and your mind. Plan your rest periods just like your workouts. Use this time to reflect on your achievements in not only the fitness aspect but also other important areas in your life. This is called passive recovery. After reading 'Rest and Recovery from Exercise' by Champion Jason Brice, you will feel more comfortable giving yourself permission to rest.

Training Principle 7: Team approach. On the elite level, some athletes are afforded the luxury of sports psychologists, sports nutritionists and an event-specific coach. Some business executives have life coaches, pastors or peers who also take an active interest in their life. You may not need a sports psychologist or nutritionist; however, you should share your journey and experience with someone. It's a great way to maintain a level of accountability. Your circle of influence should consist of those who have your well-being in mind, who understand your goals and who are supportive in every capacity.

Initially, John's ambition outweighed his talent. However, through a very methodical approach using these techniques and his ability to stay focused on his goal, John created an avenue for success. Applying these training principles to your workouts, as well as other areas of your life, will greatly enhance your level of success.

I have had the opportunity to coach or train clients from all walks of life - national caliber athletes, diabetics, physician referred, physical therapy referred, professional business people, people who work at home, middle school-aged children, adolescents with disabilities, you name it! In every case, these training principles were applied and the end results have been overwhelmingly successful!

John is not the only one who can create an avenue for success. You can too. See you at the next level.

Charmas B. Lee, ACSM HFI

Charmas.Lee@thepowerofchampions.com
719-573-6022

SECTION TWO
The Mind of a Champion

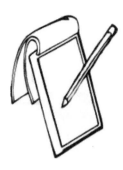

Notes from Phil

The Mind is the master of our thoughts, our actions, and at some level, our destiny. As a seed is planted, so it grows, and the mind is the garden from which thoughts are developed, cultivated, and grown into actions and achievements. While we recognize the existence of the Mind, it's difficult to define, and without a clear definition, controlling "mind-set" becomes a challenge.

Champions welcome challenge and Champion Michelle Hazlewood will begin this section by providing a perspective on balancing the intangibles, mind and spirit, with that manfestation we see in the mirror . . . the body. Champion Steven Cutler then provides some steps toward getting clear, creating a vision, and conditioning the mind to focus on the outcome you most desire. Tony Books Avilez teaches you to tune into that inner voice and he turns the partnership between self-talk and visualization into a science we can all use to further propel us toward our goals. The section concludes with Champion Chad Cirafesi identifying and helping us to master that all-powerful mind-muscle connection.

Remember Muhammad Ali chanting "I am the greatest?" His words rang with certainty. He was the greatest in his mind long before the world came to recognize his Champion status. What some might have perceived as arrogance was quite simply the greatness seed being planted. The seed was cultivated, the championship outcome an outgrowth of the implanted seed. Years before Ali wore the championship belt, Rocky Marciano said, "To win takes a complete commitment of mind and body. When you can't make that commitment, they don't call you a champion anymore."

Make the commitment. Be a Champion. Read on . . .

Balancing Body, Mind and Spirit by Michelle Hazlewood

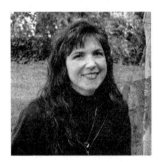

Champion Michelle Hazlewood of Thousand Oaks, California has worked in gyms, homes and corporations providing training, telephone coaching, home retreats and lectures. She has written numerous articles, contributed to wellness books and authored "Personal Success Guide for the 21st Century."

Let's journey for a while beyond sets and reps, past caloric intake and expenditure, outside exercise goals and motivation....an expedition to discover the big picture of us!

Muscles, organs, skin and bones; the Body is the area that we are most familiar with and generally focus on. We are a little less knowledgeable about the Mind, which involves the workings of our brains. But at least we have a few clues about how it functions. Most mysterious, to the general population, is the Spirit. Some refer to it as life force or the soul.

The physical body speaks loudly due to our five senses - sight, sound, taste, touch and smell. As a result, we generally spend most of our time catering to it. We eat, drink, sleep, exercise, dress and make cosmetic changes for the body.

Fortunately, we also realize the power and intricacy of the mind, so education is encouraged and ongoing research is invested in heavily. Sometimes crossword puzzles, mystery stories and other brain games are engaged in to stimulate and retain function of our brain cells.

The spirit is the most overlooked aspect of our being. Yet without it the rest of our systems are useless. Although it dynamically governs our mental and physical workings, we seldom remember its existence much less its importance.

Different camps can argue about which of the three is most essential. Let us, for the general purpose of our enlightenment, imagine a three-legged stool. All the legs must be strong and balanced for the integrity of the stool. Similarly, in our lives, the vibrant relationship of the body, mind and spirit must be attended to and nourished for our total well-being. "We live in trizophrenia – Thinking one thing, feeling another & acting a third. Sometimes we think 'yes,' feel 'no' and say, 'I'll get back to you later.'"[1] Only when we integrate body, mind and spirit throughout every day will we live in balance and harmony. So, how do we do that? How do we make the connection?

Since there are numerous resources and my fellow Champions address the body in other chapters of this book, you are already aware of the many ways to take care of yourself physically. The mind is a little more complex but, again, there is a plethora of information available and commonly known regarding its enhancement. Practices such as rehearsing, goal-setting, affirmations, visualizing and reasoning are ways the mind enhances the body's experience.

Intuition, emotion, faith, trust and love are just some of spirit's contributions. Intentionally tapping into this power source enables us to passionately live this life experience to our fullest capacities.

You have probably noticed even the medical community is realizing the importance of being balanced. Internationally renowned experts, Christiane Northrup, M.D., Andrew Weil, M.D., Deepak Chopra, M.D. and many others have all made great advancements in Integrative Medicine. This health-oriented approach takes account of the whole person - body, mind, and spirit, including all aspects of lifestyle. Emphasis is on the restorative connection and makes use of all appropriate therapies, both conventional and alternative.

Here are some modalities for you to experiment with to enhance your body-mind-spirit connection. As you play with the ideas feel which ones resonate with your intuitive wisdom and sense of values. You will come to an intrinsic awareness of the most harmonious practices for you!

- ◆ **Meditation** – Sitting comfortably in a quiet place or soft music sets the scene for some. Others enjoy a labyrinth or other walking meditation. There is no one correct way. Most people have difficulty when they first attempt to keep their mind focused in one place. That's ok, just notice extraneous thoughts and see them float away. It can be useful to contemplate a goal or challenging question. In your calm receptive state, listen for answers from your spirit's wisdom.

- ◆ **Questions** – Daily consider wisdom-evoking questions such as:

  - Are my actions in integrity with my core values and beliefs?
  - Am I honoring my inner needs as well as those external?
  - What can I do today to elevate the dynamic connection of body, mind and spirit?
  - Can I sense the dance between my body, mind and spirit in this workout?
  - How do I see my life?
  - How do I feel about my life?
  - How do I listen to what my mind and body are telling me?
  - How does my external life express my higher self?

  With each question, allow yourself to be aware of both the facts and feelings of the answers.

- ◆ **Visualization** – Many skilled athletes and other savvy professionals have now learned the power of this tool. Vibrantly picture, in your mind's eye, you performing whatever activity you would like in detail with the exact outcome you desire. Feel your movements confidently and competently flowing. Hear the unique sounds around you. Sense your emotions throughout the experience. Whether preparing for a competition or an interview, the more you practice this technique, the more amazing the results will be. Real life will closely reflect that which you specifically rehearsed.

- ◆ **Journaling** – Just the act of writing your thoughts, actions and feelings can be an enlightening exercise. It can assist you in bringing about powerful healing and positive energy. You can use the questions above to start with or just write about whatever you are sensing or feel guided toward. Other helpful themes are vision, goals, learning experiences, "*Aha*" moments and gratitude. All involve aspects of the body, mind and spirit coming together.

- ◆ **Affirmations** - With good reason, this activity has increased in popularity. Affirmations are carefully chosen, purposeful statements made frequently throughout the day and often posted in strategic locations. "I" statements, made in the positive and present, make these more effective.

  - I have a balanced connection between my body, mind and spirit.
  - I easily integrate my body, mind and spirit here and now.
  - I am at peace and harmony with my world.
  - I tap into my internal wisdom for the answers to my questions.

- ◆ **Mind-Body Exercise** – Some forms of exercise are more conducive to reinforcing the body-mind-spirit connection, such as yoga and Tai Chi. These are uplifting techniques and beneficial to many. However, once you learn the concepts of intertwining body movements and traveling deeper inside, you can apply them to other exercise modalities as well. As numerous runners will attest, getting into the 'zone' has got to be a 'mind-body' experience!

- ◆ **Conscious Living/Mindful Activity** – Usually we have so many things going on throughout the day that we are rarely "in the present." We dwell on things past that we cannot change or our thoughts race to the future worrying excessively. Our minds are a-whirr with projects, real life soap operas and what we need to do next. While it is necessary at times to multi-task, it would aid our body-mind-spirit connection to practice living consciously. Designate a time period, perhaps 15 minutes, or an activity, like running or a meal. During that time focus on all the sensations you experience. Vividly bring into play as many senses as possible, not only your five basics but your emotions and inspiration as well. The more skilled you become at this, the more you will be able to relish the deliciousness of life in the moment.

- ◆ **Make Your Choice!** - Too often we make our decisions by "should" or what we think others expect of us regardless of whether we are in congruency to what we truly believe. Try an internal self-check and start making decisions and actions by choice. Think, weigh and feel. Even if a decision is somewhat distasteful, you have the satisfaction of knowing that you have chosen it deliberately over an alternative. And when a decision brings delight that was your choice too! This empowering tool can be so freeing, leading you to greater confidence and satisfaction in your life.

These are just some ideas to start you on the dance to live a balanced life. Remember it is not a destination that you reach here but a wondrous series of movements up, down and around to reach that center where you feel whole! That is when you experience those moments when all is right with your world. Delightfully, with practice, we will reside in this place of harmonious vibrations more often.

Michelle Hazlewood, ACE

Universal Wellness
805-375-2516
Michelle.Hazlewood@thepowerofchampions.com
www.universalwellness.us

The Science of Change – Mental Conditioning by Steven Cutler

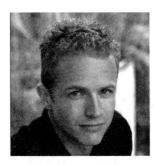

Champion Steven Cutler of Sandy, Utah is a personal fitness trainer, exercise testing specialist, natural bodybuilder, college instructor, motivational speaker and corporate consultant. He specializes in weight loss, bodybuilding, post-rehabilitative/corrective exercise, and sports performance.

Mental conditioning is paramount to your pursuit of success.

Without a strong mind you would not and could not create the body you want. A strong mind and a strong body go hand in hand. Author Sterling Sill wrote, "A healthy body is the dwelling place best suited for a clear mind, a pure heart, and an enthusiastic spirit." The strength of the body and the mind are inseparable.

Just as your body needs conditioning through specific activities and exercises, your mind needs to be trained, conditioned, and programmed to respond in positive, progressive ways. So how do you train or condition your mind for success? The following four-part plan will produce powerful results if properly understood and applied. I call it "The Science of Change™" and it will work to condition your mind and body for success. The steps are:

- Get Clear
- Get Leverage
- Get a Plan
- Get Going

Get Clear

Step one is to Get Clear. Some may call this goal setting, but it's more than that. Just sitting down and writing a goal will not guarantee you success. Getting clear is really done in two steps. The first step is what I call Reflective Clarity. Let's do this mental conditioning exercise together right now.

Get Clear Step 1 - Reflective Clarity

Find a room where you can quietly be alone with this book, a pad of paper and a pencil. Now, think back to your childhood. I want you to recall the first time you became aware of your body. What were your thoughts about it? Do you remember thinking that you were too small or too big? Did you notice a certain body part, or did someone say to you "You sure are athletic," or "You are built just like your mother?" I want you to think deeply about the first time you became aware of negative or positive thoughts about your body.

When I do this exercise with some of my clients, they tell me about experiences when they looked down at their thighs and thought for the first time, "I've got fat legs." Others remember comments or comparisons made by friends or family about their body that either made them feel comfortable or critical about themselves.

Many of the ideas we have about our bodies were shaped in our youth, and, if left unchecked, shape our success or failure later in life. Let me give you an example.

After working with someone I will call Jane for a few months she stopped progressing. Her weight loss had turned into weight gain, her progression into regression. One day I sat down with Jane and asked her to go through this exercise with me. With tears in her eyes she related to me feelings of frustration and embarrassment over her body when she was a child. She shared with me one particular story when she was younger where she got more attention than she wanted, more than she was comfortable with.

That experience made her feel like she was different, or less than those around her. She was so embarrassed about her body that she wanted to run and hide. Jane never wanted anyone to look at her body again. She associated such deep feelings of pain with getting the attention that subsequently she learned to cope with that pain by hiding her body under baggy clothes and layers of fat, while avoiding all situations where she may be recognized or stand out.

As we talked, it became apparent to Jane that this experience had shaped her image of herself in a very real way. It had altered her behavior. As she lost weight, she began getting attention. People would make comments about how good she looked and how impressed they were at her dedication. This attention caused the conditioned response of "run and hide" to manifest itself in her eating and exercising habits. She began to sabotage her success and hide behind food and fat again.

Jane, by recalling the experience, found some healing and realized that she was sabotaging her success because of the feelings or associations she had made when she was younger. Simply by recognizing what she was doing enabled her to stop the sabotage and create success. She realized that she is now a different person. She is wiser and more mature. She lost the weight that she had gained back, increased her strength, and has continued to progress ever since. Sometimes that is all it takes – recognizing why we do something - in order to change it.

Get Clear Step 2 - Create Vision

The second part of getting clear is writing down what it is you really want, and why you want it. This may sound like the same old boring goal setting, but it's not. You see, when we set goals we often do it without determining why we really want it. The key to success in any area of life, especially in fitness, is to understand why we want what we want.

Now, on your pad of paper I want you to write for the next five minutes all the goals you want to accomplish. Don't stop writing at all during the five minutes. Write down all the things you are passionate about. Create a mental vision of how you want to look and feel in the next three months. Don't waste any time – start writing!

Get Leverage

Did you do it? Good. Now, look over your list and choose three to five of the most important goals you want to accomplish. Write these goals on a separate sheet of paper with space in between each one. Now, make a line down the middle of the paper and write for five more minutes why you want to accomplish each goal. Specifically, ask yourself "What will I gain by reaching this goal? What will be the rewards?" Also, ask yourself what you will miss out on if you don't reach your goals.

Victor Frankl, author and Nazi death camp survivor, taught in his book, *Man's Search for Meaning*, that if you have a strong enough why (reason) you can live with any what (goal). Start writing your "whys" and don't stop for the next five minutes.

Great job! Now you've got some leverage. Your goals have some power behind them. They have purpose and meaning and will take on a life of their own. Remember that with a strong enough "why," you can live with any "what."

Get a Plan

You now have clear goals and reasons why you want to accomplish these goals. You're clear and you've got some leverage. Congratulations! The next mental conditioning exercise is to get a plan. Below each goal write down a deadline for each goal.

Deadlines have a very powerful way of motivating and inspiring us to move forward. Don't worry about how you will accomplish your goals right now, just when you will accomplish them by.

Next, sit down and write two to five things you need to do to accomplish each of your goals. Don't worry about getting too specific. For instance, don't say "I have to get in the car and drive to the gym, and then get on the elliptical machine and stay on there for 30 minutes, and then I have to get off the elliptical machine and go over to the leg press machine and do . . . .!" Instead write down things such as "In order to reach my goal I need to exercise on a consistent basis" or "I need to hire an expert to help me reach my goals." These are your action items. This is your plan.

Your plan may change over time, especially as you become more educated. Don't worry. It should change. One of the keys to success is altering your approach when your current approach isn't working. Einstein said, "The significant problems we face cannot be solved at the same level of thinking we were at when we created the problems." Your plan will change, you will develop a higher level of thinking, but these first few steps will create massive momentum.

Get Going

Momentum can change the outcome of an athletic event, a game, a war, a battle or your life. Look at the plan you have written and within the next 24 hours do at least one of the action items listed on your plan.

Don't let time pass before you act on at least one action item. Carry your goals with you and focus on them consistently. According to Anthony Robbins in *Personal Power*, "That which we consistently focus on over time we will create." As you focus on the above mental conditioning exercises, you will develop the mind and body you are capable of.

Remember that the strength of the mind and the body are inseparable. Develop both and you are creating change for life.

Steven Cutler, ACSM HFI, NSCA CPT

801-257-5897
Steve.Cutler@thepowerofchampions.com
www.getcutfitness.com

Mental Conditioning - Self-Talk by Tony Books Avilez

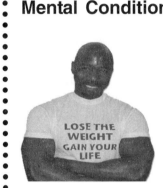

Champion Tony Books Avilez of Staten Island, New York is one of the most highly sought after speakers and trainers in the greater New York area. He is the author of 5 books on health and fitness.

In order to obtain the level of fitness and the body you want . . .

it is necessary to work.

Body transformation is surely the result of physical effort. The question is: If someone has the ability to perform the physical work necessary to be fit, why don't they? They don't because their mindset is not in alignment with the goal they want to obtain. Think about exercise and nutrition as being two cars on the same train. The engine that pulls that train is the mind.

There is an ancient ayurvedic saying: "If you want to see what someone's mind was like in the past examine their body now. If you want to see what someone's body will be like in the future examine their mind now." Everything created by human beings is the result of two births. These births are first in the mind and then in the physical world. This includes creating a new, strong, healthy and sexy body.

I'm going to share with you some concepts and strategies to assist you with a type of conditioning that you must do in order to get in your best shape ever - mental conditioning. Your mind is like a garden. Whatever you plant in it will grow. The GIGO theory is true: "garbage in garbage out." If you plant seeds of fear, doubt and indifference, that's what your future will in all likelihood become. Fortunately, the converse is also true. GIGO can stand for, "Good stuff in good stuff out." You can create a new future through renewing your mind.

The first step is making a decision. The Latin root of the word "decision" means "to cut away from." When you make a decision, you have chosen only one possible outcome. You cut yourself away from all other possibilities except the one you have chosen. This means if you have chosen to lose 20 pounds, there is no reason to even consider that you can't do it. You will find the technology that works and commit to using it to succeed. Making a decision means that you plant the seed in your mind that you will achieve your goals no matter what.

Decision and choice go hand in hand. Once you make your decision, everything else in the process involves choices you make each step of the way. These choices provide you with the power to create a new, positive and compelling future. Choice is a great thing to have, but it also comes with responsibility. Responsibility is literally your "ability to respond." With each choice, you exercise your ability to respond in alignment with your goals.

So let's talk about some strategies to strengthen your ability to respond. Positive self-talk is exactly what it sounds like. It's putting a positive spin on the conversation that goes on inside your head. To some folks this may sound crazy. You have surely been told that only crazy people talk to themselves. Well, the truth is everyone talks to himself or herself. This is simply how we think. We all make evaluations by asking and answering questions in our mind. For instance, have you ever asked yourself this question: "Should I workout in the morning or should I just wait until tonight?" When you asked that question, did you answer? Did you say in your head: "I'll just get up now and go" or "I'll sleep and go later?" If you have ever asked yourself a question and then answered it, you're crazy too! Seriously, it's crazy not to talk to yourself. Some of the thoughts that come into your mind have to be addressed - especially the ones that disempower you. You can't control all of the thoughts that come into your mind, but you can control which ones you embrace.

The perfect partner to positive self-talk is visualization. You're probably not new to the concept of visualization. This concept has been beaten to death - because it works! The process of visualization entails seeing yourself looking the way you want to look and feeling the way you want to feel in your mind first. The subconscious mind is unable to tell the difference between something real and something that is intensely imagined. You can use this either to create fear and doubt, or you can use it as a means to program yourself to reach your full potential.

Try experiencing the power of visualization. Sit or lie down in a comfortable position. Next, take five slow deep breaths holding each one for five seconds. Slowly close your eyes and release all the surface tension from your body. As you do this, create a picture in your head of the image that you want to perceive. See what your body looks like 20 pounds lighter, or whatever your ultimate goal may be. If your goal is firmer abs, picture that. Take your time and create as vivid a picture as possible. See yourself as if you are looking in a mirror at the body you want. As you continue to relax, hold on to this image and concentrate on feeling as though it exists in the present.

Next, you want to visualize your process of achievement. The same way you created the image of the body you want, see yourself performing the exercise necessary to achieve that goal. Relax and feel your body go through every repetition, every set and every workout. Feel yourself as being powerful and able to do all the work necessary. See yourself eating healthy foods every day. See yourself preparing the meals you need and eating them with enjoyment. Take time out to perform this visualization process every day and you'll find yourself becoming more motivated and excited during your transformation.

In order to speak to yourself to truly engage your mind for positive imagery and successful programming, use what is called the three P's - personal, positive and present. When you make a statement to help condition your mind for positive self-talk, make it personal. Say "I" not "you." The subconscious mind perceives "you" as being someone other than yourself.

It also does not register any negative within a positive statement. Saying "I won't miss any workouts" is not nearly as powerful as saying, "I will perform all of my workouts."

Stating your goal in the future tense dilutes the power of your statement. In other words, if you say that you want something in the future, it doesn't reinforce attaining it. Saying, "I want to lose 20 pounds" today and then saying, "I want to lose 20 pounds" in a month doesn't bring you any closer to attaining that goal in the present. Instead say "I weigh 165 pounds now!" You are claiming what you want in the present. You're telling your subconscious mind to feel that you can do it not in the future, but right now! The difference may seem subtle, but it's extremely powerful. As Champion Brian J. Johnston states in his chapter, 'Cultivating Consistency,' it's like the little stream of water that formed the Grand Canyon.

I know what you're saying, "I don't weigh 165 pounds yet. You want me to lie to myself?" No, think of it as telling yourself the truth in advance. I actually want you to stop lying to yourself. I want you to tell yourself the truth from this day forward. The truth is you are powerful, capable, resourceful, worthy and have everything you need to succeed already. You were born with it. All you need to do is tap into your God-given gifts, seek out the technology that works for you and then put it into practice. The key is to do this with a mindset of faith and maybe even reckless abandon. I urge you to train hard and say, "Yes!" to your dreams. Always remember that your journey to achievement begins within your mind.

Tony Books Avilez, CSCS

888-FIT-5186
Tony.Avilez@thepowerofchampions.com
www.thebodyhouse.com

Mind & Muscle Efficiency by Chad Cirafesi

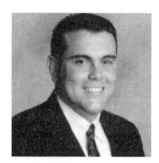

Champion Chad Cirafesi of Red Bank, New Jersey holds a master's degree in kinesiology and is about to complete a doctorate degree in sport and exercise psychology. His passion for fitness and human performance is a product of his multi-sport background and involvement in the health club and athletic industries for over 12 years.

Professionals in charge of helping us reach our maximum potential agree that the key to optimal performance is in the cultivating, fostering and encouraging of efficiency.

Merriam-Webster defines efficiency as "(1) effective operation as measured by a comparison of production with cost (as in energy, time, and money), and (2) the ratio of the useful energy delivered by a dynamic system to the energy supplied to it." To Champions, the term represents the fundamental link between desire and peak performance.

As you can tell from the chapters of this section and others throughout *The Power of Champions*, there are many different places you can seek and find areas for improved efficiency. In sports, it may be about putting a ball through a hoop, between the posts, or over the fence. In fitness, it may be about getting to the club, burning calories, or lifting weights. In work, it may be about increasing production, meeting a deadline, or turning a profit. No matter the task at hand or the goal that must be attained, making changes that create, initiate and develop efficiency is one of the clearest avenues to accomplishment.

There are many different techniques and strategies you can implement to achieve individually defined success. I will provide a general description of a few of the most effective.

Just Do It?

For many of us, making decisions about whether to take action or not, or choosing one path over another is a major barrier to making progress. While in these situations, consciously or unconsciously, we all make mental checklists of the pros and cons of making specific behavioral changes (e.g., starting a new exercise program). Performance coaches and psychologists have described this mental process as a decisional balance. Research has shown that many people do not make positive behavior changes until the perceived positives significantly outweigh the negatives. This process can serve us well, however, problems arise when the cons are based on irrational feelings and unfounded beliefs. Hence, the proper action may never be taken.

Often, we can move this process along by first writing out a list of the perceived pros and cons of taking a specific action next to each other and reviewing the completed list. Second, determine which of the statements on both sides you know to be fact and which you might consider only a belief or feeling. Finally, seek and find the knowledge needed to convert one individual belief or feeling at a time into rational statements or facts that should or should not remain on the list. You may find that taking a little time and effort to go through this simple process will lead to a much more useful decisional balance, which can lead to making positive changes and taking action sooner rather than later, saving you a lot of potential stress, guilt and resentment.

All I Need To Do Is Set Goals, Right?

We are often told that setting goals is essential for better performance; however, very rarely do we set performance-based goals. Too often, we define our participation in life in terms of success and failure or winning and losing. For some, this black and white approach to goal setting can be motivating. For most, unfounded notions about perceived consequences create deep pitfalls and large speed bumps on the path to peak performance. Rather than worrying or speculating about the consequences of victory or defeat, a Champion concentrates on the steps that must be taken to perform better the very next time their mind and body is called into action.

A performance goal can be based on general measures such as how many times you exercise in a week to specific measures such as the tenth of a second you shave off of a race time. These goals do not need to be tied to a particular measure but can also focus on the performance of a specific behavior (e.g., keeping your head down on the next golf swing), which will lead to better performance through repetition. No matter what the task, the performance-evaluation-adjustment-performance cycle is more efficient with performance goals that are not based on competition with others as much as with oneself. In this paradigm, setting smaller short-term goals serve as the building blocks of progress toward attaining long-term accomplishments. Progress becomes the root of motivation instead of perceived negative consequences. Champion Jonathan Ross' chapter, 'Excellence – A Culmination of Tiny Steps,' really drives home the importance of small steps leading to big results.

Mind & Muscle

For Champions, the mind and muscle link is one of the most powerful avenues for improved efficiency and performance. Often, our mind gets in the way and works against us rather than being the driving force for change and efficiency. Somewhere between establishing goals and making steady progress toward these goals, our heads can become clouded by negative thoughts, stress, and over-thinking. Cognitive restructuring and tension /anxiety regulation are methods you can utilize to combat this breakdown and promote peak performance. To learn how to recondition your mind, read 'The Science of Change – Mental Conditioning' by Champion Steven Cutler and 'Mental Conditioning – Self-Talk' by Champion Tony Books Avilez.

Many cognitive restructuring techniques (e.g., Self-Talk, Rational Emotive Behavior Therapy, Positive Affirmation, etc.) focus on the ability of emotions resulting from our thoughts to effect behavior. Aside from promoting positive self-talk, many interventions seek to help us cope with undesired consequences and dispute or replace the negative thoughts that lead to unproductive emotions. Here is an example of how the thought-to-emotion-to-behavior chain can be restructured:

John is about to play in his first collegiate game next week. He keeps playing the following statement in his head, "If I lose, I will be letting down my team and everybody back at home." Based on the potential consequence of losing, he is already experiencing guilt, anger and shame that can lead to undesired anxiety and tension. By analyzing this statement and disputing its rationale, John is able to revert to thoughts such as, (1) "If we lose, it will be because the team didn't perform well," (2) "Playing at this higher level of competition will be a great learning experience, and (3)"Those that love and support me back home will know that I tried my best."

Anxiety and tension regulation can often be categorized as either mind-to-muscle or muscle-to-mind. Autogenic and visualization techniques are ways of using our minds to help our bodies reach optimum anxiety and muscle tension levels for the task at hand. Autogenic training includes the learning through practice of progressively inducing feelings of weight or warmth in the desired muscle groups to promote relaxation and reduce muscle tightness. Visualization techniques can help a person to simulate real life situations and match prior peak performances. We mostly hear about visualization in relation to sport participation but the technique can be used in many other areas such as fitness (e.g., body image), education (e.g., test taking) and the corporate world (e.g., presentations).

Breathing and progressive muscle relaxation techniques are ways of using our bodies to help our minds reach optimum anxiety and muscle tension. Aside from exhalation and inhalation rates, many breathing techniques focus on promoting the best ratio of nasal vs. mouth and diaphragm vs. chest breathing. Progressive relaxation includes learning to systematically create tension in one to all muscle groups in the body to induce a natural tension reduction response. This overall reduction in tension can, in turn, allow your mind to focus on the desired task.

Summary

Peak performance is dependent upon our ability to make good decisions, make progress along individually defined performance goals, and make the mind and muscle connection work for us rather than against us. There are many types of interventions that can promote this sort of efficiency. However, respect must be given toward the inherent ability of our mind to learn and adapt from situations in the past and allow our bodies to perform at their optimal levels in the future.

Chad Cirafesi, M.S., CSCS

732-687-8142
Chad.Cirafesi@thepowerofchampions.com

SECTION THREE
The Body of a Champion

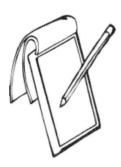

Notes from Phil

At the age of 14, Ian Thorpe became the youngest male swimmer ever to find a place on the Australian Swim Team, and in 1998, at 16, he won the 400 meter freestyle World Championship making him the youngest male World Champion in swimming history. He's amassed a slew of Gold Medals and broken swimming records every year since. Ian was quoted as saying, "People ask me 'what was going through your mind in the race?' and I don't know. I try and ...let my body do what it knows." The connection between mind and body should now be clear. In the previous section, we discussed the mind. Now it's time to move to the physical manifestation, the body. Just as Ian Thorpe trained his body to gain performance knowledge, you are making progress along a road to your body just "knowing" excellence.

Champion Dan Houston begins the section by taking the mystery out of a word everyone knows, but few really understand, Metabolism. Champion Eric Anderson then explains the framework and provides you with the power to maintain and improve the skeletal system. You'll join Peter Piranio for a compelling discussion about the tissue that allows the skeletal system to move and learn about the correlation between muscle tissue and metabolism.

We'll then turn to Champion Amy Powlison to help you make certain that if weight loss is a goal, the weight that you lose is fat weight, allowing you to preserve the lean body mass that drives the metabolic machine. With an understanding of body composition, Champion Lisa Martin will continue on the topic and educate us in the area of determining precisely what our pounds are made up of.

Champion Bryan Lanham will open your eyes to some of the characteristics that make us unique and he'll empower you to match an exercise routine with your specific body type. This exciting section ends with Champion Jason T. Hoffman opening your eyes to some of the less-recognized, perhaps shocking, "other" benefits of exercise.

One of the most powerful tools in assessing physical change is a preliminary photograph. As you acquire the information shared by the Champions, you become further empowered to facilitate positive change. The photographs act as evidence to the gradual improvement that allows you to ultimately love your reflection, and the greater ease with which you move through life serves as testimony to the fact that as you learn, your body will "just do what it knows."

Understanding Metabolism by Daniel Houston

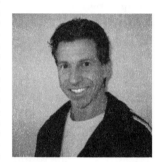

Champion Dan Houston of White Lake, Michigan and his wife, Cherie, own Houston Fitness Consultants, a private training studio. Using their unique "Chile Pepper Approach," 12 years combined experience, and common sense, they make training entertaining, effective, functional, efficient and educational.

We often hear from clients that they think they have a "slow metabolism."

It is beneficial to make sure they understand what "metabolism" means and how lifestyle and exercise choices may affect their ability to reach their body composition goals.

What is metabolism? It is all the reactions that take place in the body that involve the transformation of energy. It is the process of combining nutrients with oxygen to release the energy needed to function. Metabolic reactions are either anabolic or catabolic. Anabolic reactions require the addition of energy, such as building muscle and bone; catabolic reactions release energy, usually by breaking larger molecules into smaller molecules. Every movement, every reaction requires energy. The total expenditure of these reactions is measured in kilocalories, which we refer to as calories. This number is the total energy requirements of your individual metabolism.

The largest percentage of total metabolism is RMR, or Resting Metabolic Rate. This typically represents 60-75% of the total metabolic rate. We refer to this as "the minimum amount of energy required to maintain the machine."

Additional metabolic demands come from the thermic effect of food, which is the amount of energy required to digest the food consumed. This can account for about 10-15% of the total. Champion Kelly Huggins discusses the thermic effect of food in greater detail in his chapter, 'Burn Fat by Eating More!'

The balance of your body's caloric needs comes from activity level, which is the easiest variable to manipulate. We can directly increase our need for energy by increasing our activity levels. Done correctly, we can create a calorie deficit that will require more efficient fat assimilation to resolve. Resistance training can increase the "value" of lean mass, resulting in slightly higher post-exercise oxygen consumption and reduced breakdown of lean tissue to supplement calories.

RMR represents, in calories, the daily amount of energy required by your body to sustain the metabolically active tissues while in a resting state. The number is used to represent average daily calorie requirement, based on sixteen hours sitting still and eight hours of restful sleep. This does not always accurately represent a person's RMR, however. Certain situations can affect RMR including fever, overtraining, poor sleep, illness, obesity, certain medicines, supplements, poor digestion, restricted calorie diets, rapid weight loss, etc. All of these must be taken into consideration.

There are a couple of commonly used methods for determining approximate RMR. Trainers routinely use the ACSM guidelines, body composition and activity measurements. Dietitians have used the Harris-Benedict Equation, using height, weight, age, and gender. These formulas have limitations; we have seen them off by 18-25% with some clients. They are still considered fairly accurate for most people. The most accurate method we have encountered is using an indirect calorimeter to measure actual oxygen consumption. It gives an accurate baseline, with consistent, repeatable results.

Lean mass is the highest percentage of RMR. Lean mass is more than just muscle. It is all metabolically active tissues and systems in the body, including the central nervous system, respiratory, vascular, endocrine, digestive and lymphatic systems. Bones, too! All systems require energy, in varying levels, to be maintained. What happens when the caloric consumption is below their RMR for an extended period of time? A reduction in system efficiency! All the systems need to be fed! Even stored adipose tissue requires some energy. Consistently consuming less than RMR will result in a reduction in lean mass, reduced digestive efficiency, reduced performance, slower recovery, hindered immune system function, restless sleep, hormonal imbalance, and a higher risk for injury.

This is often seen in low calorie diets. Below RMR, the body makes lean tissue available to supplement caloric deficit. The loss of lean tissue results in a lower RMR (less mass to feed) and reduced metabolic functioning. Extreme low calorie eating does not necessarily use fat to make up this deficit. Instead, lean tissue is sacrificed because it is an easier conversion, requiring less energy. It also lowers RMR to closely match intake. The result of this is a new RMR which may be low enough that normal eating patterns will result in large calorie surplus, potentially quick weight gain, primarily as body fat. Lean mass generally does not increase unless the skeletal muscles are stressed sufficiently to require it (as through resistance training).

Adding up RMR, the thermic effect of food, projected activity level, and body composition goals can give you a daily calorie target. When you know what you need to have, you can plan to make the most of your eating. We know that there are thermic benefits to eating smaller, more frequent meals. It is also easier to digest, and more efficiently absorbed. Most people can efficiently digest 500-700 calories at a time. Eating more calories than that at one sitting is similar to putting thirty gallons of gasoline in a twenty-gallon tank. It is a waste of fuel, a waste of money, and it is bad for the environment (in this case, adding to stored body fat). The same thing applies to food. If it is not necessary, it is easier to not eat it than to try to work it off later! Something to think about: before your body starts to burn fat, teach it not to store more!

Large meals require more blood and energy for digestion, which will leave the body feeling lethargic and tired. Less blood and energy is available to the limbs and muscles, which will result in a decrease in activity. Activity is the best way to increase your metabolic requirements. Daily activity accounts for about 10-20% of your metabolism.

Eating based on your body's need for food for a given time period makes for efficient meal planning. For example, someone needing 2400 calories per day to meet their metabolic needs could easily figure 400 calories per meal, at six evenly spaced meals per day.

Since it is not practical to eat exactly the same amount per meal, we recommend that our clients try to make their meals provide fuel proportionate to their need for fuel. Metabolic rates are lower when we sleep, higher upon waking, and can be sustained at an elevated level by trying to eat based on need. An easy meal plan is to provide for three meals, with dinner being slightly lower in calories than breakfast and lunch to match the normal decline in metabolism toward evening, and three snacks to maintain energy requirements and lessen the tendency to overeat at the next meal. Healthy food choices are important! If the body is going to go to all of the trouble to break down the food for fuel, it should benefit from the compounds and micronutrients supporting the calories.

Applying an automotive example, think of food as fuel for your daily journey. It would be easier if we could just put all our fuel for a long trip into the car at once. We could drive without stopping! Unfortunately, we have to plan for our fuel stops because we know we can only go a set amount on a tank of gas. Too little fuel, we end up on the side of the road. Since we cannot put in more fuel than our tank will allow, we have to accept the limitations of the design.

It is the same with eating for fat loss. It would be easy to just eat one meal for the day, addressing all our total energy needs, and force our body to burn fat for the remainder of the day. Unfortunately, it does not work that way! We have to provide enough fuel to take care of the daily activities, the detours, and occasional side trips. The best way is to not waste fuel, and plan ahead. Use enough to get to your destination, and enjoy life along the way. Eating just enough to maintain an anabolic environment promotes better fat assimilation, and reduced fat storage.

We offer metabolic testing at our private studio as an accurate method of establishing individual RMR. This small, non-invasive test gives our clients valuable information for maximizing their exercise and eating for weight management. The small expense for the test is easily offset in less wasted time and wasted food. We encourage our clients to enjoy their food but recognize it as fuel for the body. Feed it!

Total metabolic requirements determine fuel demand. Add to that personal goals, exercise tolerance and recovery ability, and a plan can be developed that will work for everybody.

Dan Houston, ACE CPT/LWMC, NFPT

President
Houston Fitness Consultants
2624 S. Milford Road
Highland, MI 48357
248-676-2882
Dan.Houston@thepowerofchampions.com
www.houstonfc.com

The Skeletal System and Exercise by Eric Anderson

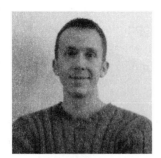

Champion Eric Anderson of Champlin, Minnesota is a personal trainer in the Minneapolis, Minnesota area who, through proper health and fitness instruction, teaches people how to unlock their true potential and inspires them to live life more abundantly.

The skeletal system is the one system of the body that seems to be most often neglected when it comes to discussing and/or implementing an exercise program.

Everyone seems to be more interested in discovering the fastest, most effective way to add muscle mass, shed unwanted body fat, run faster, throw farther, jump higher, or just look good in a bathing suit. Yes, these are all admirable goals indeed, but let's not forget one basic principle: Without the skeletal system, none of these things would be possible! No one would look good as a blob of tissue lying on the floor, no matter what he or she is wearing.

The skeletal system is composed of approximately 206 bones and more than 300 joints. Simply put, it is a system of levers and hinges that work together to provide the framework for the body's structure and function.

In order for the skeletal system to do its job efficiently, it must be able to maintain proper alignment. Each bone has an ideal, predetermined position, and the muscles attached help keep them in line. Every move you make is dependent upon the location of each specific bone and its ability to move in a desired direction with the least amount of resistance. All of the bones that make up your skeleton need to be in the right place at the right time in order for your body to function optimally. The term used to describe this position is posture, a word we all heard growing up but seem to have forgotten somewhere along the way.

Webster's definition of the word posture is "the relative disposition of the parts of something." Regarding the human body, it simply means where your bones are in relationship to one another. By the way, sit up straight! Your body requires more muscles to be activated in the slouched position, which I'm sure you are in right now, than it does to maintain good posture.

Proper posture reduces pressure on joints, increases available energy, makes you more comfortable, improves your attitude and gives you more self-confidence. It allows your body to evenly distribute the forces that are being placed upon it at all times and in all directions. Whether it's the incessant force of gravity pulling you toward the earth or a barbell stacked with a challenging amount of weight, your body has to be able to spread the force evenly. Without proper alignment, your body learns to function sub-optimally by altering its support structure according to the parameters set by the newly designed center of gravity.

Sound confusing? Humor me for a moment. Let's compare your body to the body of a car. If the wheels are out of balance or the alignment is off, the tires begin to wear unevenly in an attempt to correct the problem. Over a prolonged period of time, the car starts to pull to one side or the other and begins to vibrate once it reaches a certain speed. More effort is then required by both the driver and the car to drive straight. The car is no longer operating at maximum efficiency. Get the picture?

Your body responds in a similar fashion. If your skeletal system is not lined up properly, by default, your muscles, like the tires, must attempt to compensate. Your frame is then pulled to one side or the other and tiny vibrations start to occur. Stiffness and soreness soon follow, and life - as you know it - is no longer the same. In other words, you become the "pain in the neck" for everyone else around you. You complain about how you feel and talk about the everyday tasks you used to do with ease that you no longer can because it hurts to do them. And, even if you could, you just don't have the energy. Sound familiar? Sit up straight! I'm sure you're slouching again. It's a never-ending battle. Now do you understand why posture is so important?

In the words of Sir Charles Sherrington, "Posture follows motion like a shadow. All movement begins and ends in posture." It is the foundation from which all activity, or movement, is derived, not just another reason for your mother to scold you and smack you upside the head. After all, body mechanics, the way in which your body moves, is nothing more than the study of posture in motion. Let's take a closer look.

When you decide to make a move, your brain has to communicate with your muscles through a system of nerves in order for a series of muscle contractions to take place. The muscles, which are attached to various bones, are then able to provide the body with the movement necessary to complete the desired task. If, however, your body detects a problem anywhere along the way, it must immediately develop an alternate route so that the assignment can be completed. In essence, if someone is out of line or not pulling his or her fair share of the weight, someone else has to step in and pick up the slack. This leads to a change in the pathway, which is the beginning of a chain reaction that throws the body's entire movement pattern out of whack. Believe me, it's not pretty. And, it can be quite painful. But it doesn't have to be this way.

A combination of strength training and stretching, on a regular basis, can prevent a traumatic experience like this from ever happening to you. Strengthening the right postural muscles and making sure that your program is designed to include opposing muscle groups will give you the strength and stability needed to maintain proper alignment.

Several studies have shown that strength training also helps to increase bone density, which is one of the many things we struggle to maintain as we get older. Approximately 10 million Americans suffer from osteoporosis, a condition defined by the National Institutes of Health as "a skeletal disorder characterized by decreased bone strength, with a predisposition to an increased risk of fracture." The fact of the matter is this number will undoubtedly increase during the next 5-10 years as the "baby boomers" begin to reach the age of 60. The less active you are, the greater the chances are that you will eventually suffer from osteoporosis as well. With a proper diet and exercise routine, however, your risk can be greatly reduced.

Throughout life, bone growth occurs at a fairly steady rate. By the time you reach your mid-twenties, your bones are as dense as they're going to get and have achieved what is called peak bone mass. At this point, your bones reach the top of the mountain, structurally speaking, and they pretty much hang out there for the next 20-30 years. Eventually, however, all good things come to an end, and the process of bone loss begins. But the speed at which it takes place can be altered.

Just because bone growth ceases at a certain age doesn't mean they are no longer active. Your skeleton actually continues to replace itself at the rate of about one-fourth of its structure per year. It does this by incorporating two different types of cells, osteoclasts and osteoblasts. Osteoclasts, the demolition crew, come in and remove old bone so that the osteoblasts, the construction crew, can come in and install the new bone, thus completing the remodeling process. It's a bit more complicated than that, but you get the basic idea.

According to Wolff's Law, one of the primary factors in determining where and how much of this remodeling takes place is exercise. The law states that the amount and strength of bone are directly linked to the amount of activity that forces the bone to bear weight and move against resistance. Therefore, participating in proper weight-bearing exercises, like strength training or running, allows your body to become more structurally sound and reduces the risk of developing osteoporosis in the future.

No matter what your reason is for wanting to start an exercise program, I hope you are beginning to see that all aspects of your life are ultimately affected. Every system in your body operates more efficiently. The less energy you spend on the simple tasks, the more energy you'll have to spend doing the things you love. Exercise helps you to reverse the past, enjoy the present, and look forward to the future!

Eric Anderson, NASM CPT

10928 Utah Ave North
Champlin, MN 55316
(612)423-9377
Eric.Anderson@thepowerofchampions.com

A Concern for Muscle by Peter Piranio

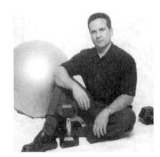

Champion Peter Piranio of Milwaukee, Wisconsin is owner of Piranio Fitness Systems, Inc. and Fitness Together in Delafield and Brookfield, Wisconsin. He received his bachelor's degree in Fitness Management and Business Administration from Carroll College in Waukesha, Wisconsin.

A Concern for Muscle - If you don't have it – you better get it!

What would you do if I told you I have the secret to long-lasting-put-a-smile-on-your-face-weight-loss and it would only require 5% of your day?

What if I told you physicians prescribe it to lower cholesterol, offset the effects of osteoporosis, turn back the clock and reverse years of physical neglect?

What if I showed you how it will burn fat while you are watching TV, lying on the beach, and even when you're sleeping? Not to mention it will also allow you to eat pizza or ice cream every once in a while!

Finally, what if I said it is the absolute key to changing your body and the only side effect is your bathroom scale may not work anymore?

Ten years ago I would have probably guessed you would have yelled: How can I get some and how much is it? But today, I would bet you are pretty skeptical and may have already written me off. I can't blame you. With the proliferation of fad diets, metabo-mumbo-jumbo, and fitness gimmicks people just don't know what works and what doesn't. To make it even worse, huge companies are stealing your money and abusing your trust by promising impossible results if you just drink their shake, take their pill, or do 10 minutes of exercise on their wiz-bang machines all in the name of profits and market share.

All skepticism aside, trust me when I say you can have long-term fat loss, change your body, improve your health and even burn fat while you sleep all by having a concern for muscle. Hold on, don't shut the book yet! Let me explain. Having a concern for muscle simply means increasing or at least maintaining your current lean muscle weight. That's it. Pretty simple, don't you think? Maybe we do have some obstacles that make this a little more challenging. But I do want to be clear here, the other components discussed in *The Power of Champions* play a vital role and when put together produce the results I am promising.

First of all, let me start by easing your concern about the side effects. I told you that it will have an effect on your bathroom scale, but don't worry. If it's brand new, take it back. Most stores will refund your money. If it has become part of your family and you wake up to "Mr. Scale" every morning, just politely ignore him. Let's face it, he has not been kind to you and most of the time gives you the first bad news of the day. If you are not that sentimental, just throw it away because the scale is really not that smart. As a matter of fact, it is psychologically self-defeating.

If it is fat loss you are seeking, you must first understand that it is body composition that really matters, not the scale. Ideally, if you have a concern for muscle, you would like to increase your body's lean muscle. Ladies, don't worry, I don't mean bulking up. You could easily increase your lean muscle by five pounds and still lose inches. If you increase your lean muscle by five pounds, lose five pounds of fat and your jeans feel loose, what will the scale say? It will say you weigh the same. So you have to make a decision, do you care what the scale says or how your jeans fit? My fellow Champion, Amy Powlison, states the facts with regard to weight in the next chapter, 'Fat Loss Rather than a Focus on Pounds.'

Now that I have eased your concerns and stomped out one of the biggest myths and obstacles to your success, let's talk about a vital component of having a concern for muscle – incorporating resistance training.

Having a concern for muscle requires you to stimulate the muscle to a point of momentary muscle failure. This momentary muscle failure produces a stimulus that creates an adaptation by your body – an increase in lean muscle! This is exactly what you want and yes, even if you want to lose a hundred pounds, you want more muscle. The vehicle through which you create momentary muscle failure and an increase in muscle is resistance training.

The biggest mistake I see people make is buying into the notion that dieting and aerobic exercise is the solution to achieving weight loss. To make matters worse, there is the belief that resistance training does not burn fat. Nothing could be further from the truth. In fact, resistance training is probably the most misunderstood and underrated component to fat loss and body transformation. It is critical to lasting fat loss.

Why is it so important? One word - metabolism. You are in control of your metabolism. We often think we inherit our metabolism and there is nothing we can do about it. Wrong! Having a concern for muscle plays a vital role in increasing your body's utilization of calories. As Champion Dan Houston explains in his chapter, 'Understanding Metabolism,' three factors contribute to your total energy expenditure - fueling the resting metabolic rate (RMR), the thermic effect of food and voluntary activities. Here is the most important part! Your metabolism is proportional to your body size and lean mass.

That means an increase in muscle will increase your RMR, or the amount of calories your body requires to sustain its existing state. So, if at a bare minimum you consume the same amount of calories and have more muscle, you will create an energy debt. This debt will result in body fat loss. But the metabolic benefit of resistance training does not stop there. An added bonus is the temporary increase in metabolism after a resistance training workout. It is estimated that for those forty-eight hours after a workout your metabolism will be temporarily elevated to aid muscle recovery.

But wait there's more! Fat oxidation, or the burning of fat as energy, takes place in the muscle. If you have more muscle, what do you think that does for your ability to burn fat as energy? That's right, you just made yourself a much better fat-burning machine! Ladies, this pertains to you as well. Please be sure to read Champion Kelli Calabrese's chapter, 'Fat Burning Secrets for Woman.'

Muscle is metabolically active tissue. Fat is not. Fat is an energy source for the body, but it uses very little energy. Muscle uses energy. Lots of it! As a matter of fact, each pound of lean muscle tissue burns 35-50 calories a day whereas body fat only burns about 2 calories a day. The bottom line - the more lean muscle you have, the more fat you burn even while at rest.

Do you have a concern for muscle yet?

You see, that's really the key to long-term-put-a-smile-on-your-face-weight-loss. Looking great is not just a function of how much fat you burn when you're working out, because you can only exercise so much in a given week. The real secret is how metabolically active your body is the other 95% of the time. People with more lean muscle burn fat at a much greater rate than those with less. That doesn't mean you have to look like Arnold Schwarzenegger. But you do have to at least maintain and preferably increase your lean muscle tissue. Have a concern for muscle and you will achieve the body transformation you desire.

What this all boils down to is making the personal commitment to change and holding yourself accountable.

Peter Piranio, B.S., CSCS

262-646-5444
Pete.Piranio@thepowerofchampions.com
www.piraniofitness.com
www.fitnesstogetherbrookfield.com

Fat Loss Rather than a Focus on Pounds by Amy Powlison

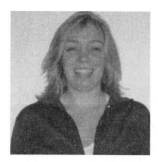

Champion Amy Powlison of Philadelphia, Pennsylvania offers an energetic and empathetic approach that makes fitness fun for her clientele, which ranges from S.W.A.T. members, athletes, and 400 lb. clients.

Time and again I hear members, clients, and friends talk about losing weight.

But for successful weight loss, there are several questions you need to ask yourself in order to develop realistic and attainable goals.

Why do you want to lose weight?

What type of weight do you want to lose?

What do you weigh?

What is your percent body fat?

You would not buy a car without researching it first. Similarly, you should not try to make changes to your body without doing the same. This chapter will arm you with the information you need to make informed decisions, enable you to set achievable goals and successfully change your body.

What is percent body fat?

What "is" body fat, for that matter?

Percent body fat is the measurement of what percent of your weight is adipose tissue, commonly known as fat. Everyone needs a certain amount of fat to live. Body fat lines organs, helps regulate body temperature, and is the body's main form of energy storage.

The following table contains the ranges for various categories of body fat.[2]

Body Fat Percentage		
Categories	Women (% fat)	Men (% fat)
Esssential	10-12%	2-4%
Athletes	14-20%	6-13%
Fitness	21-24%	14-17%
Acceptable	25-31%	18-25%
Obese	32% and higher	25% and higher

Obesity is defined as a high percent of body fat and is a serious health risk, which requires immediate attention. Changes in nutrition and exercise will usually reduce body fat to the acceptable range. If you fall within the acceptable range, your goal should be to reduce body fat to the fitness category. Knowing how percent body fat relates to overall health will help you understand why it is important to be conscious of body fat reduction rather than weight loss.

In addition to being in better shape, other health benefits exist for individuals who have a lower percent body fat. Serious excesses in body fat place a person at higher risk for diseases and other conditions, including diabetes, high blood pressure, heart disease, high triglycerides, high cholesterol, and joint problems, to name just a few. In addition, if you are carrying most of this excess weight around the waist, you are at an even greater risk for developing these conditions. A lower percent body fat decreases the occurrences of developing these diseases and conditions. That is not to say a lower percent body fat guarantees that you will not develop any health problems. However, maintaining a healthy body fat percentage significantly lowers your risk, further confirming the importance of percent body fat and the need to concentrate on losing fat, not simply 'weight.'

When someone begins an exercise program and makes nutritional changes, it is quite feasible that their body fat may decrease while their weight remains the same. In order to understand how this is possible you must get rid of the idea that muscle weighs more than fat. Not true! A pound is a pound is a pound. One pound of muscle does not weigh more than one pound of fat any more than one pound of rocks weighs more than one pound of feathers. Muscle is denser than fat so by volume it weighs more yet takes up less space than fat.

For this reason, it is important to focus on your percent body fat rather than the number on the scale. When weighing yourself on a scale, you weigh every part of your body's makeup, including skin, muscle, bones, organs, fat, and all the rest. There is no separation between your lean weight, or fat-free mass, and fat. Lean mass and some fat mass are required to live. Why weigh yourself at all then? Because your weight helps determine more valuable information, including your percent body fat. By recording your weight at the start of your weight loss program, you establish a baseline for future reference.

After making informed decisions and acting on those decisions to change your body, your weight and body fat can be rechecked and compared to your previously recorded baseline to determine progress. Looking at scale weight does not clarify if you even need to lose weight and, if so, how much. Using percent body fat shows what weight can and should be lost to increase health. For example, a 140 lb. female with 30% body fat decides her goal is to lose 30 lbs. Using the following equation, let's see if this is a realistic goal for her.

Equation	Body weight x percent body fat = # of pounds of fat
Body Fat	140 lbs. x 0.30 body fat = 42 lbs. fat
Lean Mass	140 lbs. – 42 lbs. = 98 lbs. lean mass
Weight Loss Goal	140 - 30 lbs. = 110 lbs.

If she loses 30 lbs., she would have 98 lbs. of lean weight and only 12 lbs. of fat or 11% body fat. This goal falls within the essential range for women, which is not realistic to achieve and would be very difficult to maintain.

A better way to determine her weight loss goal would be to decide what body fat percentage she would like to achieve. Let's use 22% as an example, which falls within the fitness range for women.

Body Fat	140 lbs. x 0.22 body fat = 31 lbs.
Goal Weight	98 lbs. lean body mass + 31 lbs. = 129 lbs.
Weight Loss Goal	140 lbs. – 129 lbs. = 11 lbs.

A loss of 11 lbs. is a much more realistic, achievable, and maintainable goal in this case.

This can be a hard concept to accept. Getting on the scale and deciding your health according to your weight is ingrained in our heads from childhood. Everywhere you turn media, magazines, friends, and family all have an opinion on weight. Mainly, the lower the number, the healthier, happier, more successful, and beautiful you should be. Focusing on body weight alone develops unrealistic expectations, which can lead to disappointment, bad eating habits, poor workout regimens, or taking extreme measures. Stop! Do not set yourself up for failure. The number on the scale is not that important. Refocus! Start looking at percent body fat over everything else. To find out how to determine your body composition, read Champion Lisa Martin's chapter, 'Measuring Body Composition Effectively.'

Which brings us back to the question I posed earlier: What type of weight do you want to lose? Hopefully now you see how this loss in weight should come from a concentration of fat. If not, you still need to work on removing old ideas from your mindset and replace them with more accurate information.

Look again from another angle. Which man is healthier and in better shape - a man who weighs 200 lbs. with 41% body fat, or a man who is 200 lbs. with 18% body fat? The man who has 18% percent body fat is much healthier than the man with 41% body fat.

Who is healthier - a man who is 200 lbs. with 18% body fat, or a man who is 170 lbs. with 32% body fat? Do not be misled by weight. It may surprise you, but the man who weighs more is healthier and in better shape. By revisiting the equation from earlier, this becomes evident.

Body Fat #1	200 lbs. x 0.18 body fat = 36 lbs.
Body Fat #2	170 lbs. x 0.32 body fat = 54.4 lbs.
Difference	54.4 lbs. of fat - 36 lbs. of fat = a difference of 18.4 lbs. of body fat

The man who weighs less is actually less healthy because he carries an additional 18.4 lbs. of fat on his body.

Hopefully, the concept of concentrating on fat loss not weight loss is making sense. You should now be able to answer my initial question: Why do you want to lose weight? Before you may have had general answers like to look better, feel better, etc. Now you should know how to turn those answers into more specific goals. You do not just want to lose weight. You want to lose 5 pounds of fat to decrease your body fat to 20% in order to increase your overall health, and decrease your risk of developing numerous health conditions. Now that is a goal!

Whatever your reasons for wanting to lose weight, make sure to determine what that term really means, and develop realistic and specific goals to ensure your success. Good luck!

Amy Powlison, NSCA, R.A.D., AFAA

215-873-4572
Amy.Powlison@thepowerofchampions.com

Measuring Body Composition Effectively by Lisa Martin

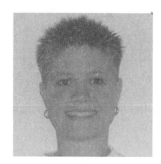

Champion Lisa Martin of Columbia, Maryland holds B.S. from the University of Maryland in Dietetic. Her company, Focused Fitness, conducts seminars and personal training for school and corporate programs, individuals and small groups.

As a society, we are more out of shape and unhealthy than ever before.

It is rare to go somewhere and not hear or see information on how to lose weight. We frequently use weight loss as a major indicator of successful (or unsuccessful) fitness efforts. So, what is wrong with using your weight as a measurement of progress? As Champion Amy Powlison discussed in the previous chapter, focusing on weight rather than body composition leads to unrealistic goals and ultimately failure and frustration.

How can you begin to look at and evaluate your program differently and more effectively? It's time to become more educated and learn how to accurately measure your results.

Weight is defined as the vertical force exerted by the mass of an object as a result of gravity. How does this relate to your health since it does not explain the exact makeup of the object? On the other hand, body composition measures the percentages of muscle, fat, bone and other tissue that make up the body. Body composition takes total body weight and breaks it down into more detail by separating the body into adipose tissue, or fat mass, and lean body mass, or fat-free mass. It is expressed as a percentage of body fat to total body weight.

First, realize that body fat is present for a reason. It acts as insulation, regulates body temperature, cushions joints, protects organs, fuels the body, aids in reproductive function and stores vitamins. For these reasons, among others, your body fat will never be zero. Women carry more body fat than men partly due to the reproductive responsibilities of the female. This difference in males and females is first noticed during puberty. From this point, men show a lower body fat percentage than women. Along with aging comes a natural decrease in lean body mass and a slower metabolism making it more difficult to lose body fat.

In order to lose body fat, your body must burn excess stores through a process known as thermogenesis. Thermogenesis occurs when your body produces heat through metabolically active tissue. Brown fat is thought to be more metabolically active fat tissue and is important in the breakdown of storage fat. Storage fat is known as white or yellow fat. It is more inactive and functions as cushioning for your organs and an insulator for your body. Currently, studies are looking at the impact of brown fat on obesity. Many people think cellulite is also a type of fat. Cellulite is actually a cosmetic term for fatty deposits under the skin separated by connective tissue. When these fat cells increase in size, it creates the appearance of dimpling in the skin. From a biochemical standpoint, cellulite is no different than normal body fat.

So, how then do you determine your body composition? There are many different methods available for estimating body composition but only cadaver studies are completely accurate. Since most people don't prefer an autopsy, there are other options! Realize that the available methods only measure within a range of accuracy. The most common methods to measure body fat are:

- underwater, or hydrostatic, weighing
- skinfold calipers
- bioelectrical impedance

Hydrostatic weighing is considered the "gold standard." This method is probably the most expensive and the most inconvenient of all methods.

Skinfold calipers are an accurate alternative to underwater weighing. The American College of Sports Medicine has shown caliper measurements to be up to 98% accurate when compared to underwater weighing. These measurements are taken at various sites on the body and, for the most part, give a pretty accurate view of fat distribution. Additionally, they tend to have the least amount of variation from measurement to measurement provided you have an experienced tester. When using body fat for evaluation purposes, improvement is more important than actual body composition numbers. Skinfold measurements accurately show improvement.

The process for determining body fat using calipers is very simple. All measurements are taken on the right side prior to exercise. For women, measurements are most commonly taken from the middle of the arm over the triceps, just above the hip bone known as the iliac crest, and the front of the middle thigh. The chest, abdomen just right of the belly button and the front of the middle thigh are used for males. Depending on the chart, some other commonly used sites may be subscapula on the bottom point of the scapula, the widest part of the inside of the calf and just below the armpit at the midaxilla. Using a chart, your age and the sum of all the skinfold sites, your body fat can be determined.

Bioelectrical impedance measures the body's resistance to an electrical current. It is based upon the premise that the conductivity of an electrical impulse is greater through lean mass than fat. The analyzer places electrodes on the wrist and ankle. For accurate measurements, you should be well hydrated, avoid exercise for at least 6 hours prior and have consumed no alcoholic beverages for at least 24 hours. Research has shown this method to be as accurate as skinfold measurements provided the test is done correctly. It is fast and easy but can be expensive, ranging from $300 to $5,000.[3]

If you do not have access to any of the above methods, you can still track your progress. One of the easiest methods is to take girth, or circumference, measurements at various sites on the body. For these measurements, you only need a cloth or vinyl flexible measuring tape, like those used by a tailor. The measurement sites are: upper arm at the widest point between the shoulder and elbow; your waist at the smallest point above the belly button; hip measurements at the widest part of the buttocks and thigh measurements at the midpoint of the upper leg. These measurements are best used to show loss in specific places. Although you cannot spot reduce, this will allow you to see a bigger picture of what is going on over time.

Now that you know your body fat percent, how do you know what is considered a healthy range? The average healthy range for women is 21–24%. The lowest a woman should strive for is 14%. A healthy recommended range for men is 14–17%. Men should go no lower than 6%. Obesity is classified by body fat percentages of 32% and higher for women and 25% and higher for men. In this case, risk for disease is extremely high. Due to the insulating role of body fat, you may see a slight increase in the colder winter months.

If your body fat measurements do not fall within the healthy range, you can change it by, you guessed it, changing your eating habits and incorporating strength training and cardiovascular exercise into your daily routine. Cardiovascular exercise burns calories, even hours after activity. Think of cardiovascular exercise as any activity that increases your heart rate to a level that you can sustain for an extended period of time. Strength training creates a greater increase in muscle mass, which increases your overall metabolism. Strength training is any movement that involves using resistance to build muscle and develop strength. Resistance bands, dumbbells, Nautilus machines, body weight, and water are all tools that can be used for strength training. Increasing lean body mass through exercise and decreasing body fat means your body can burn more calories, even while at rest. This will help you decrease your overall percentage of body fat.

In order to grasp how and why body composition is more effective, you must first understand why weight can be misleading. Measuring weight accurately is sometimes very difficult as it naturally fluctuates depending on when and where you take your measurements. This is not to say you should not know your weight, but use it as an additional tool and measure it periodically. Your degree of progress will certainly depend on your starting point. Additionally, when you focus solely on weight loss, you risk losing a lot of water weight and lean muscle in the process. This will only create a fat skinny person, someone within his or her healthy weight range with a high percentage of body fat.

When setting goals for your specific fitness program use body composition as your main measurement. Make a commitment to yourself to change your current lifestyle. Do it for your health and your future. Once you make the commitment, take small steps to develop lifelong habits, not temporary quick fixes. To set reasonable goals, measure your starting body composition, determine your desired body composition then set your long-term and short-term goals.

Take it one step at a time, prioritize and stay focused on what is important to you. Realize that it has taken years to get to your current condition so patience is the key. Give it time and work hard - results will happen!

Lisa Martin, B.S.

410-707-0055
Lisa.Martin@thepowerofchampions.com
www.focusedfitness2000.com

Sizing Up Exercise: Training Different Body Types with Different Routines by Bryan K. Lanham

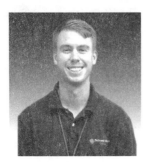

Champion Bryan K. Lanham of Danville, Kentucky is a Wellness Counselor and Personal Trainer at McDowell Wellness Center in Danville, KY. He holds the Certified Strength and Conditioning Specialist (CSCS) credential from the National Strength and Conditioning Association (NSCA).

Results are important to everybody, but every body is different.

A one-size fits-all approach to fitness doesn't work. The following will address and explain specific information that should be taken into consideration when designing and implementing individualized training programs.

Have you ever wondered if you could look like your favorite pro athlete if you really got serious about fitness? The answer to this question in one word is genetics. Athletes such as Michael Jordan and Arnold Schwarzenegger were blessed with genes that were conducive to attaining superstardom in their respective sports of basketball and bodybuilding. The majority of us will never "be like Mike" or compete for the titles of Mr. Olympia and Mr. Universe, but we can make the most out of what we've got. While there are natural limitations to the amount of muscle you can pack on your frame, everybody can build muscle, no matter what your age, sex, or body type.

In the 1940's, Dr. William H. Sheldon introduced his widely accepted system for classifying body types. His theory states that there are three main body types – endomorph, ectomorph and mesomorph. Below you will find a description of and recommended exercise prescription for each type to help you get the most out of your workouts.

Wrist girth is a good determination of body type. Wrap your left thumb and middle finger around your right wrist. If your fingers overlap you have a small frame and are an ectomorph. If they just touch you have a medium frame and fall into the mesomorph category. If your fingers don't touch you have a large frame characteristic of endomorphs. Once you assess your body type you can customize your training to maximize results.

Endomorph

People in this category have a slower metabolism, are generally shorter, have medium to large frames, and have the genetic predisposition to put on fat easily. These are the people that seemingly gain weight by just looking at food. In order to keep percent body fat within the recommended range, endomorphs should diet and exercise appropriately.

Exercise Prescription:

Since endomorphs tend to carry more body fat, their workouts should focus on burning calories. Cardiovascular exercise should be longer and more frequent. Try to do some cardio most days of the week. Be regular and consistent and don't worry about working at a high intensity starting out. Excessive pounding is hard on the joints of heavy-set individuals. Aim for 20-30 minute sessions at a moderate intensity in your Target Heart Zone (THZ). Increase the amount of time by one or two minutes each workout until you are doing 30-45 minute sessions. After a month, you can zigzag your cardio sessions by staggering high and low ends of your THZ. Another name for this is interval training. For example, work for 30 seconds to one minute at 80-85% of Maximum Heart Rate (MHR) followed by 1-2 minutes at 65-70% of MHR. Cardio sessions such as this should be done for 20-30 minutes or 8-12 intervals. Champion Brett Pruitt explains the ins and outs of target heart zone in his chapter, 'Putting Your Heart into Your Exercise Program.'

Strength training is equally important for the endomorphic body type because building muscle raises your metabolism. Since muscle is more metabolically active than fat, you burn more calories throughout the day, even at rest. For more on the metabolic benefits of muscle, check out Champion Peter Piranio's chapter, 'A Concern for Muscle.'

Total body circuit training with high reps, supersets, and exercises is recommended for endomorphs. A circuit is a group of exercises performed consecutively. Supersets, as described in the Introduction, work opposing muscle groups back to back. You can train protagonist and antagonist muscles such as back/chest, quadriceps/hamstrings, biceps/triceps, and low back/abs using this principle. Choose one exercise for all of the major muscle groups and move from one exercise to another with little to no rest in between. Shorter rest periods (30 seconds maximum) help elevate your heart rate to elicit a more aerobic effect.

Exercise larger muscle groups first because if you pre-fatigue smaller muscles you won't be able to work the larger muscles as efficiently. Beginners perform 1 set of 15 reps for each exercise in the circuit. Use a weight that is challenging and brings you to the point of momentary muscular failure. Intermediate exercisers perform 2 circuits of 15 repetitions per exercise for each pair of movements with 1-2 minutes of rest in between circuits. Advanced exercisers perform 3 supersets of 8-15 repetitions per exercise for each pair of movements, increasing the weight slightly for each consecutive circuit. Endomorphs should strength train 3 times a week, every other day.

Diet tip:

Consume fewer empty calories. Empty calories come from foods high in saturated fat and sugar. Read the chapters in Section 6 on 'Eating Like a Champion' for the information you need to fuel your body for fitness.

Ectomorph

Ectomorphs have smaller frames and faster metabolisms. Their extremities are usually longer and they exhibit a slim build. Their high metabolism allows them to burn fat easily and maintain lower body fat percentages. The downside to such a metabolism is that it is difficult to gain and maintain muscle mass, therefore ectomorphs are known as "hard gainers."

Exercise Prescription:

Cardiovascular exercise should be less frequent and done at a light to moderate intensity. Prolonged bouts of cardio are detrimental to the muscle building effects of weight training so do no more than the minimum recommendation of 30 minutes in your THZ, 3-5 times a week.

To maximize muscular development ectomorphs should lift heavier weight and perform fewer repetitions using compound movements, such as squats, that work multiple muscle groups at one time. In his chapter 'Reducing and Shaping Your Hips and Thighs,' Champion Darrell Morris describes compound exercises and their benefits. Ectomorphs should workout at a slower pace, allowing adequate recovery time between sets and workouts. Perform 1-3 sets of 6-10 repetitions resting 1-2 minutes between sets. Never work the same muscle group twice within a 48 hour period. Larger muscles like the legs should be rested longer between sets. If you are a beginner, start with one set and increase as tolerated. Pyramid the amount of weight used with each successive set by starting with a weight that you can perform 10 repetitions, on the next set add 5-10% to that weight and do 8 repetitions, etc. Remember to use a challenging weight that takes you to the point of momentary muscular failure within the prescribed rep range.

Diet tip:

Increase caloric intake and never skip meals. Eat six healthy meals a day. Consider supplementing your diet with multivitamins, amino acids, creatine, glutamine, and protein shakes to aid muscle recovery and fuel muscle growth.

Mesomorph

Mesomorphs are blessed with athletic, naturally muscular physiques. Mesomorphs exhibit a medium to large frame. They have the advantage when it comes to building muscle rapidly because they are genetically predisposed to do so. They also tend to lose fat rapidly when on the correct diet. It would seem that people with this body type have everything going for them. While this is true to some extent, they too must watch their diets and exercise regularly to be physically fit.

Exercise Prescription:

Moderation is the key for this body type. Since mesomorphs are less prone to store an excessive amount of body fat, aerobics shouldn't be done as frequently. Three days a week at a moderate intensity in your THZ should suffice. Like endomorphs, mesomorphs can include interval training in their cardiovascular routine. Weight train all of the major muscle groups with moderate to heavy resistance. A basic weight routine of 3 sets of 8-12 reps with moderate to heavy resistance is recommended. Rest about 1 minute between sets and 1 day between workouts. You will gain lean muscle more quickly than the other two types.

Diet tip:

Eat a nutritious, well-balanced diet of "clean" foods including lean protein and complex carbohydrates to maintain your lean, muscular build. Section 6, 'Eat Like a Champion,' provides excellent guidelines for making healthy choices to support your fitness regimen.

Remember, you cannot change your body type. Accept the fact that you are what you are and train appropriately. The information I have given you will help you get the most out of what God gave you, not morph you into something you're not. Vary your routine every 4-6 weeks to break the monotony and prevent your body from acclimating to your workouts. Changing variables such as frequency, intensity, time, and type of exercise prevents overtraining and plateaus.

Bryan K. Lanham, CSCS

McDowell Wellness Center
1107 Ben Ali Drive
Danville, KY 40422
859-936-WELL
Bryan.Lanham@thepowerofchampions.com

The Other Benefits of Exercise by Jason T. Hoffman

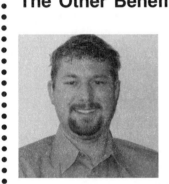

Champion Jason T. Hoffman of Lowell, Arkansas has a background in exercise science with an emphasis in athletic training. He works as an exercise physiologist in a medical facility focusing on the non-surgical treatment of neck and back injuries.

Exercise, or physical activity, has been defined as "bodily movement produced by skeletal muscles that results in energy expenditure."[4]

It is clear that a certain level of physical activity will result in a person achieving physical fitness, or, in other words, being physically healthy both externally and internally. Some obvious external benefits to exercise include weight loss, muscle gain and body reshaping. Obvious internal benefits include improved flexibility and muscular strength, increased endurance and metabolism and more efficient conditioning of the heart.

There are numerous other benefits to exercise that are not as obvious. These benefits involve the "internal" physiological and psychological improvements that develop within a person, all of which are derived from physical activity. We will explore some of these other, more obscure, benefits to exercise that, although not exhaustive, will certainly be eye-opening and should motivate you to incorporate an appropriate exercise program into your routine.

For one, physical activity slows the progression of osteoporosis, a degenerative disease of the bones that causes the bones to become brittle and more prone to fracture. There is no "best treatment" for osteoporosis, other than preventing its occurrence in the first place. The disease affects 10 million Americans, most of them women, but an additional 18 million Americans also have osteopenia, or low bone mass, that increases the risk for osteoporosis. Since bone mass increases during puberty and reaches its peak between ages 20 and 30, it is important to begin an exercise regime as early as possible and maintain an appropriate program throughout your adult life. Weight-bearing exercise, which is the best type of activity to prevent osteoporosis, applies tension to muscle and bone, and encourages the body to compensate for the added stress by increasing bone density by as much as 2% to 8% a year.[5]

There are two ways in which exercise is beneficial to the health of individuals with diabetes. First, exercise uses glucose, or sugar, in the blood for energy, which lowers blood glucose levels. Diabetics who can achieve a more constant level of blood glucose require less insulin injections, which can lead to greater enjoyment of life. Second, exercise stops the blood vessels in the heart from expanding, which helps prevent heart disease - - the leading cause of death for diabetics.[6]

Exercise benefits the body by stimulating the nervous system. The increased workload of exercised muscles results in an increased metabolic rate, and calorie (or fuel) consumption, which causes a person's internal body core temperature to increase. This increase acts as a stimulant to many parts of the body, including the glands, muscles, nerves, joints and circulatory system.

Exercise also affects the endocrine system, which regulates the natural hormones in the body. Specifically, the glands respond to exercise by releasing certain hormones that lower cholesterol, elevate mood, suppress appetite, and aid in digestion, among other things. The stimulating effect on internal body temperature, combined with the release of certain hormones resulting from exercise, can and often do, provide significant relief for those who suffer from certain mental health problems. These hormonal changes act on specific areas of the brain that control pleasure and elation. In fact, a recent survey found that 83% of people with mental health problems looked to exercise to improve their symptoms. Two-thirds said exercise helped to relieve the symptoms of depression and more than half said it helped to reduce stress and anxiety. Some people even thought it had a beneficial effect on manic depression and schizophrenia.[7]

The cognitive system is also positively affected by exercise. Similar to the endocrine system, the nervous system is stimulated during physical activity. As the core temperature increases, the nervous system and the nerve-muscle communication become more efficient. These changes affect specific areas of the brain increasing alertness and, possibly, intelligence. Further, decreased tension caused from physical activity can also result in better sleeping patterns, which would further aid in alertness and cognitive retention.[8]

Exercise improves lymphatic flow and increased immune-system resistance. The lymphatic system, the body's second circulation system, is an important part of the body's defense against disease and toxins. Movement of the lymphatic fluid toward the heart is partially dependent on muscular compression of the lymphatic vessels, which are strengthened from exercise. Exercise results in a general improvement in bodily function, combined with improved lymphatic flow and increased immune hormonal balance.

There are several other psychological benefits to exercise. After a certain amount of physical activity, we have a feeling of well-being, the stimulated nervous system is more alert and, as a result, we tend to display more confidence. The increased energy level, combined with increased glandular output, results in improved energy levels and increased sexuality, stamina, and resistance to fatigue.

Physical activity stimulates the body and its natural peristaltic function, involuntary muscle contractions that assist in the flow of bodily contents in digestion, which can lead to regularity in waste elimination. Exercise also aids in intestinal function by giving the digestive organs a healthy tone. The strength and conditioning that exercise provides can also assist in preventing problems associated with stomach hernias and ulcers, which can occur from weaknesses in the muscle and surrounding tissues.

Exercise lowers cholesterol, a type of "fat" present in the blood, which leads to an improvement in circulation. Some studies at Stanford Medical School have shown that moderate dietary changes, combined with aerobic exercise, can improve cholesterol levels and, thus, lower a person's risk for developing coronary artery disease.[9] Aerobic exercise is best for lowering LDL, or "bad cholesterol," and raising HDL, or "good cholesterol" levels. However, it can take up to a year of sustained exercise for HDL levels to show significant improvement.

The best way to prevent coronary artery disease is to burn a minimum of 250 calories a day (the equivalent of about 45 minutes of brisk walking or 25 minutes of jogging). Moderate exercise alone reduces the risk of heart attack, but sustained physical activity is needed to raise HDL levels. Resistance training offers a complementary benefit by reducing LDL levels. Triglycerides, which are the chief form of fat in the diet and the most common form of fat stored in the body, are raised after a high-fat meal. Triglycerides can be lowered either with a single, prolonged aerobic session or by several shorter sessions throughout the day. Two significant ways to increase physical activity are to use the stairs and to park as far away as practical from the location you are visiting whenever possible.

Putting an increased load on a muscle through exercise causes the muscle to increase and become stronger and shapelier. The connective tissue in the muscles becomes stronger, and the muscle-nerve interaction improves. This can result in improved physique, grace, coordination, balance and posture, which will affect a person's natural body language. Also, the increased blood flow and oxygenation caused from physical activity give your skin a natural, healthy glow, which may also have a positive effect on your self-confidence.

High blood pressure is sometimes referred to as the "silent killer" because it has no signs or symptoms, yet it is a major risk factor for stroke, heart disease, and kidney disease. More men than women have high blood pressure in their early and middle years, but it becomes an increasing problem for women once they reach menopause. Physical activity can lower blood pressure, thereby increasing mortality. Many recent studies have shown that regular aerobic exercise over several months may modestly lower blood pressure. According to a recent National Institutes of Health conference, aerobic exercise reduces resting blood pressure in people who have hypertension by an average of 11 points off the systolic reading (top number) and 9 points off the diastolic (bottom number). These results could be sufficient to lower a person's high blood pressure to within normal range.[10] For more information on the benefits of strength training for individuals with hypertension, please see Champion Wayne Westcott's chapter, 'Strength Training and Blood Pressure – The Heart of the Matter.'

All in all, physical activity has a significant impact on reducing obesity and disease, and, ultimately, mortality rates. However, insofar as exercise has been linked with increased intelligence, alertness, sexuality, self-esteem, mood and mental health, an increase in physical activity may also heighten quality of life. You may have weight to lose when you begin your exercise program, but you have much more to gain as well.

Jason Hoffman, B.S.

308 Greens Cove
Apt. 206
Lowell, AR 72745
479-443-4441
Jason.Hoffman@thepowerofchampions.com

SECTION FOUR
Train Like a Champion

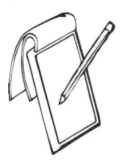

Notes from Phil

As you already know, resistance exercise is a vital piece of the physical change puzzle. By this point, as you're beginning to develop the attitude of a Champion, you no doubt believe you can find great benefit from your weight training program. But Champions know not only what they're capable of, they also know what lines they shouldn't cross. While curling dumbbells can do wonders for the biceps, attempting to curl an uprooted tree can do more harm than good. In this program, most of you will not be curling trees, and for those who aspire to such a bizarre goal, the Champions will urge you to take the necessary precautions.

Whether you're lifting stones or challenging 5 pound dumbbells, you're going to want to understand a bit more about the body which is why we begin this section with Champion Jim Beatty explaining how you can judge whether your training intensity is adequate. We follow with Champion Erik Naclerio's advice on remaining injury free.

As you progress through this section, you'll continue to amass information leading you to greater levels of understanding of and mastery over your own body. To help you gain clarity, Champion Heath Gay will zero in on the definitions of "aerobic" and "anaerobic" exercise, two commonly used but rarely understood terms. Champion Clint Phillips will share the importance of avoiding that crippling "plateau" by focusing on the value of the endless search for a new stimulus.

Champion Todd Scott will shed some light on the idea of training to get those "perfect abs" everybody seems to want and Champion Mark Cibrario will help you see the difference between what might have been deemed "conventional resistance exercise" and real world movement that revolves around human function. Champion Juan Carlos Santana reinforces Cibrario's teachings by explaining how optimal exercise approaches break away from those standard movements which we've traditionally seen in health clubs. Champion David Thomas follows on the theme of functional training by revealing some of the techniques world class and recreational athletes alike can benefit from. Champion Matt McKinnis then discusses the type of training that has helped him improve performance in adventure racing and can lead to yet a new level of physical excellence.

Champion Carter Hays introduces a method of (get ready, big words ahead) Neuromuscular Stabilization Training. It may sound intimidating, but it really involves training muscles in a manner that enhances balance and stabilization. Staying within the realm of unconventional but highly effective training techniques, Champion Stephen Holt reveals the Routine That Worked Wonders.

Champion Brian Schiff concludes the section by sharing a training ideaology that prevents stagnation and allows you to keep progress ongoing.

By the time you complete this section, assuming you read only one chapter per day, not only will you begin to note some evidence of physical improvement, but you'll be fully prepared to continue your exercise program knowing it's effective, efficient, and result oriented for the rest of your long, healthy, and fulfilling life!

Intensity & "Undertraining" by Jim Beatty

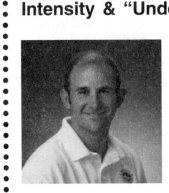

Champion Jim Beatty of Collegeville, Pennsylvania has been involved in the fitness industry since 1993 and services a clientele ranging from professional, collegiate, and high school athletes to those with orthopedic injuries, heart conditions, and neurological disorders.

In-ten-si-ty

1. extreme degree of anything

2. great energy or vehemence, as of emotion

3. in physics, the amount of force or energy of heat, light, sound, etc.

For our purposes, this definition should also be added to Webster's Dictionary:

4. in training, the amount of effort one exerts, physically, mentally, etc.

Intensity is one of the basic principles of exercise, and also one of the most important when it comes to getting results. When designing an exercise program, either for yourself or someone else, certain principles need to be addressed. These principles are:

1. **Intensity** – how hard you exercise
2. **Duration** – how long you exercise
3. **Frequency** – how often you exercise

There are numerous other variables to consider, but these are the big three. How long you exercise (duration) and how often you exercise (frequency) are going to be determined by how hard you exercise (intensity). These three principles are forever "married" and one cannot be addressed without consideration for the other two. It has been said that you can either work hard, or you can work long, but you cannot work hard and long.

The proper amount of intensity can, and should, be applied to strength training (anaerobic), cardiovascular training (aerobic), and the overall attitude with which one approaches training (including nutritional habits, sleeping patterns, etc.). Basically I'm talking about not cutting any corners.

In every strength training program, there is a level of intensity (or effort) below which little or no strength gains can occur. As with any stress, and exercise is stress, the principle of Progressive Overload must be strictly adhered to. Progressive Overload states that in order to increase the strength and/or size of a muscle, it must be stressed, or overloaded, beyond its present capacity. This means that you must ask your body to do more than it is used to doing.

Let me back up a step, and talk a little bit about exercise as stress, because I'm sure some of you are thinking, well, exercise relieves stress… how can it be stress? Exercise is only exercise because that's the name it has been given. Just like a dog is only a dog, because we (humans) have given them that name. Same for cats, toasters, treadmills, etc. Exercise is the term we have designated for bodily exertion (stress) for the sake of health. Exercise and its benefits are just another example of the process of stress adaptation. In fact, it's a perfect example of the body's ability to adapt to whatever it is presented with. Let's dig a little deeper, shall we?

Getting a suntan is an adaptation to stress. Exposure to the sun's ultraviolet rays is the stress, and from that exposure the body will release more melanin into the skin to ward off future attacks of those rays (stress). Too much sun (stress), our skin burns, peels, and we've lost all adaptations. Same with exercise. Too much, we overtrain and lose all training effects. Too little sun (stress), there is no reason for the body to adapt, and the skin will remain as pale as ever. Too little stress in exercise, no reason for the body to adapt, and we'll remain as weak and unhealthy as ever. This is the focus of this chapter: What is that necessary and optimal amount of stress?

Just like each of us has a different tolerance to the sun, we each have a different tolerance to exercise and intensity of exercise. By choosing our parents wisely, we each have been given a genetically predetermined amount of recovery ability. Unlike our tolerance to the sun (predetermined amount of melanin in the skin), we can actually have an active role in improving our tolerance to exercise by improving our recovery habits - nutrition, sleep, stretching, etc. If you're pale, you're pale. That's it. Load up on the sunscreen.

Focusing on the recovery process can absolutely improve your exercise tolerance and allow you to reach the pinnacle of your genetic capabilities. And since more time is spent recovering than training, each of us should approach our recovery with the same amount of intensity with which we approach our training. In his chapter, 'Rest and Recovery from Exercise,' Champion Jason Brice guides you through the rest and recovery process.

Okay, enough analogies… Do you understand the simple and logical principle of progressive overload? Overload the systems in a progressive manner. It is simply the process of stress adaptation.

There are several ways in which the intensity of training can be increased.

- Add more weight
- Do more repetitions
- Add more sets

- Decrease your rest time
- Change the speed of the repetitions (slow down or speed up)

Any one or any combination of the above variables will be perceived by the body as more stressful and will result in a specific adaptation. This is known as the SAID Principle - *S*pecific *A*daptations to *I*mposed *D*emands. Your body will adapt specifically to whatever demands are placed upon it.

Be sure to increase the intensity of your training by small increments. Any amount of improvement in weights, reps, etc. will be recognized by the body as more stressful, although it may not be perceived by the mind to be any more difficult. Be careful not to reach too far, too soon. Oftentimes those with the best of intentions will overreach and then subsequently overtrain. Overtraining is a state that can sneak up on you quickly when you're not paying attention as you will learn from Champion Sandy Rusch in her chapter, 'Overtraining – When Exercise Becomes Too Much of a Good Thing.'

Undertraining, however, is a state that is all too comfortable, which is why many people are sucked into it daily. The mindset of "doing something is better than doing nothing" is a very dangerous one. While it may be true on some level, thoughts such as this allow us to waste time, stagnate, and even backslide. Going through the motions… be it an easy set of 10 reps on a chest press, or an easy walk on the treadmill… is not very productive, and certainly not efficient.

If you set aside a certain amount of time out of your busy schedule to go to the gym or go for a run, shouldn't you make it as productive as you possibly can? Training with the proper intensity will assure that time spent on yourself, for yourself, is as effective and efficient as possible.

I am not advocating training at the highest intensity possible all the time. Training, to be effective, has got to be cycled. It must include periods of high intensity, moderate intensity, low intensity, and periods of no intensity. One way, as evidenced in Champion Clint Phillips chapter is to always look for a new stimulus. Time off is not a bad thing. Time away from training will allow both the body and the mind to fully recover from the stress that is placed upon them. Time off will make you "hungry" again.

What I am advocating is training at the proper intensity necessary to achieve your desired goals. There is a fine line between training with too little intensity, the proper amount of intensity, and too much intensity. This is a line that is also different for everyone, so don't look to anyone else to tell you what the right amount of intensity is. The only way to determine what the right amount of intensity is for you is to keep accurate records (weight, reps, sets, rest, time, distance, heart rate, body composition, etc.) and monitor your progress. As long as you continue to progress, chances are you're doing something right. When progress stops, look at the possible reasons why. Are you not training hard enough? Are you training too hard? Are you not getting enough rest? There are a lot of variables to consider. Not sure how to determine your target heart rate zone for cardiovascular activity? Champion Brett Pruitt takes you through it step by step in his chapter, 'Putting Your Heart into Your Exercise Program.'

Lance Armstrong recently said, "Time is limited, so I better wake up every morning fresh and know that I have just one chance to live this particular day right, and to string my days together into a life of action and purpose." Now that's intensity!

He is absolutely right. We have but one chance to make the most of what we've been given. The ability to train to improve our bodies and our minds is both a gift and a challenge. May we all have the strength, will, and courage to approach our lives and our training with the same type of intensity.

Train smart!

Jim Beatty, B.S., CSCS/CPT, NSCA

Berwyn Squash & Fitness Club
610-888-8898
Jim.Beatty@thepowerofchampions.com

Injury Free Resistance Training by Erik Naclerio

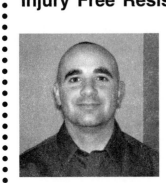

Champion Erik Naclerio of Randolph, New Jersey is the owner of Trainers Edge 1 to 1 Fitness Studio located in Denville, New Jersey. He holds a B.S. degree in Exercise Science/ Kinesiology and is a Certified Nutrition Specialist with 11 years of training experience.

"Keep your abs tight!" "Exhale – Don't hold your breath!" "Bend your knees!"

Why are statements like these being spoken by trainers around the world? No, it is not to sound like an overbearing parent watching over their firstborn. Rather, they are used to provide safe and effective exercise techniques to their clients. Lifting weights can be fun and extremely gratifying, yet there are inherent risks. The good news is that through proper education and exercise technique, these risks can be minimized. Using proper exercise technique is the most effective way to avoid injury in the weight room.

Goal Setting

Your training goals will depend on your physical maturity, age, gender and purpose, i.e., sports conditioning, post-rehab, or prevention of osteoporosis. You will need to consider the mode (type of exercise you will use), the frequency (how often you will do each exercise) and the duration (how long your training session will last). Once these goals have been determined, it is time to step into the weight room and warm up.

Warm Up

A proper warm up should be specific to the sport or activity you wish to participate in. It begins with a general warm-up period, which may consist of 5-10 minutes of walking, slow jogging or riding a stationary bicycle. The warm up increases your heart rate, blood flow, deep muscle temperature, respiration rate, viscosity of joint fluids and perspiration.[11] A warm muscle exhibits a greater amount of flexibility, so it is important to perform an activity-related stretching routine before hitting the weights. The duration of a stretching routine should last 8-12 minutes. Stretch to a point of discomfort, not pain. Increasing flexibility will be minimal if pain exists. Rather, damaged muscle or connective tissue would be the end result. To avoid injury during the stretching phases of your warm up, perform static (non-ballistic) stretches and hold each for 10 – 60 seconds. Static stretching is easy to learn and extremely effective. Do not bounce or hold your breath while stretching.

Now that your body temperature and joints are warm, it is time to minimize the likelihood of injury through prudent risk management.[12] Perform one or more warm-up sets with relatively light weights, concentrating on the shoulders, knees and back. This will stimulate blood flow to the muscles effecting the movement, increasing the temperature and pliability of ligaments, tendons, and other structures.[13]

All exercises should be performed in a slow and controlled manner. Never let gravity or momentum dictate the movement of the exercise. By moving slowly through a full range of motion, a muscle will work at a greater capacity, thus minimizing the chance of injury. Any pain felt around the joints should not be taken lightly. 'Working through' pain will only lead to chronic injuries. If pain is severe and persistent, eliminate or temporarily suspend all lifting that affects the injured joint. For example, while performing a pushup, you notice an uncomfortable feeling in your shoulder joint. The pain persists several days after your workout, however, you do not want to miss your next scheduled training session. Instead of pushing your limits on this injured area, workout your lower body and allow your shoulder time to heal. Remember, work around the injured body part.

When Pain Occurs

If you do experience pain or discomfort while performing an activity, stop the activity immediately. More often than not, the discomfort you are feeling is caused by improper exercise technique. This is the time to ask a certified fitness professional for help. He or she will evaluate your technique and correct your form. Improper form may produce a minor strain on a muscle, tendon or ligament. This is not a serious problem. However, as previously mentioned, 'working through the pain' will eventually cause more trauma to the injured area making a once acute injury chronic.

Paying close attention to your exercise technique is very important to avoiding injury. As with any physical activity, there is a degree of risk involved with resistance training. There are two specific areas that are more prone to resistance training injuries - the lower back and shoulders.

Low Back Injuries

Back injuries can be extremely debilitating, constant and difficult to cure. Most spinal disk herniations occur at the disks between the lowest two lumbar vertebrae (L4-L5) or between the lowest lumbar and the top sacral vertebra (L5-S1).[14] This is not surprising given the high compression forces on these disks during lifting.

Implementing the following three rules into your daily lifestyle and training regimen will greatly reduce the chance of injury.

> **Rule 1:** Avoid all unsupported forward flexion. – Bending over from the waist with straight (locked) knees and picking something up off the floor is unsafe. The back muscles operate at an extremely low mechanical advantage and, as a result, the muscles must exert forces that frequently

exceed ten times the weight lifted. Always bend your knees and lift with your legs when lifting something off the floor.

Rule 2: Keep your abs tight! – Whenever you perform an exercise, the abdominal muscles must be able to create intra-abdominal pressure. This occurs when the diaphragm and the deep muscles of the torso contract generating pressure within the abdominal cavity. This aids in supporting the spinal column during lifting. Such support may significantly reduce both forces required by the erector spinae muscles to perform a lift and the associated compressive forces in the disks. [15, 16]

Rule 3: Always have soft knees! – A common mistake most people make when lifting is keeping their knees locked. By keeping the knees slightly bent, the spinal column will be able to maintain its natural S-shaped form, thus providing little damage to the vertebrae, disks, facet joints, ligaments and muscles of the back.

Champion Katie Mital's chapter, 'My Aching Back,' provides additional guidelines and tips for avoiding or overcoming low back pain as well as exercises and stretches to keep the low back strong.

The Shoulder

Extreme ranges of motion and weak rotator cuff muscles are two primary reasons why shoulder joints can become inflamed and irritated. Strength training exercises such as behind-the-neck lat pulldowns and military shoulder presses place substantial loads on the shoulder muscles. From an injury prevention and muscular development standpoint, it is imperative to pull the weight toward the top of chest (slightly below chin level) during the lat pulldown.

The same can be said for the military shoulder press. Place the weight in front of the body and do not allow the elbows to bend more than ninety degrees. The following rules should apply anytime you strength train the shoulders and upper back.

Rule 1: Eliminate all behind-the-neck motion. - This may eventually cause shoulder impingement and rotator cuff damage.

Rule 2: Strengthen the rotator cuff muscles (supraspinatus, infraspinatus, subscapularis and teres minor). - These four muscles make up the foundation of the shoulder joint and are instrumental in keeping the ball of the humerus in place.

Rule 3: Avoid extreme ranges of motion. - According to Frank Jobe, M.D., co-director of the Kerlan-Jobe Clinic, "Reaching your arms too far backward on a pectoral contraction is risky. At the farthest point, the shoulder joint is not supporting the muscles anymore – only tendons and ligaments. With pressure of heavy weights, you risk rotator cuff injuries."[17]

General Precautions

Here are some do's and don'ts that should be incorporated into any strength training program for maximum safety and effectiveness.

Do's

- Use spotters when you try any unfamiliar movement.
- Breathe out during the exertion phase of the movement.
- Keep the natural S-curve of your spine during lifting.
- Emphasize correct technique.
- Make sure equipment is well maintained.
- Give your muscles enough time to recover (at least 48 hours) between workout sessions.
- Balance your muscle groups.

Don'ts

- Don't hold your breath or hyperventilate when you lift heavy weights.
- Don't use gravity or momentum as assisters when lifting.
- Don't attempt maximal lifts without proper preparation.
- Don't let your knees bend more than ninety degrees on any weight-bearing movement, i.e., lunges, squats, leg extensions and leg curls.
- Don't work a muscle group on two consecutive days.

The bottom line is to make educated decisions when it comes to your fitness program. All exercise routines should be individualized and catered to your goals. Workout at your own pace and never sacrifice proper form and technique for a few more pounds or an extra rep. The benefits of a properly designed and executed program are well worth the efforts. Work hard, work safe and enjoy the rewards.

Erik Naclerio, B.S., ACE, CSCS

Trainers Edge Inc.
Denville, New Jersey
973-627-2070
Erik.Naclerio@thepowerofchampions.com

The Two A's of Exercise Success by Heath Gay

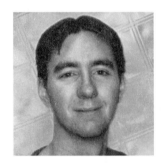

Champion Heath Gay of Colorado Springs, Colorado is the owner of Rocky Mountain Fitness Services in Colorado Springs, Colorado. He holds a bachelor's degree in kinesiology and certifications in personal training, group exercise instruction, and post-rehabilitation.

There is an expected outcome or result for everything we do.

Exercise is no different. Some people want to lose fat, others want to build muscle. All of us want to be healthier and feel better about ourselves. The question is what type of exercise will get you the results you want?

You have two choices - aerobic and anaerobic exercise. Aerobic means "with oxygen." Typically, aerobic exercise is dubbed cardiovascular, or cardiorespiratory, exercise because the heart, lungs, and blood vessels work together to achieve a training effect. Walking, running, bicycling, swimming, stair stepping, cross-country skiing, and using an elliptical machine are examples of aerobic exercise. The term anaerobic means "without oxygen." Resistance training, also known as weight lifting or strength training, is the best example of anaerobic exercise because the high intensity and short duration required to stimulate muscle growth doesn't require oxygen.

The words aerobic and anaerobic actually refer to the systems the human body uses to provide energy for every activity that goes on both inside and outside of your body. Where does the energy your body needs come from? You guessed it! Food supplies energy in the form of the nutrients carbohydrates, proteins, and fats. Fats yield the highest energy potential by providing 9 calories per gram, with carbohydrates and protein giving up 4 calories per gram. Once ingested, each nutrient is broken down into its usable form. Carbohydrates turn into glucose (sugar), fat into free fatty acids, and protein into amino acids. The energy we get from these nutrients is then turned into a usable compound called ATP. Are you bored yet? Stay with me, it will be worth it. I promise.

There are three energy systems your body uses to tap into ATP. The first two systems do not need oxygen for energy production and so are anaerobic. The third energy system does require oxygen and is therefore aerobic. Here's a crash course in how it works in your body. Intense muscular activity lasting around 15 seconds uses ATP that is already present in the muscles along with another substance called phosphocreatine. After the first 15 seconds or so, this energy system is depleted and muscles must rely on glucose (from carbohydrates) for energy. After a couple of minutes of continuous activity, the body shifts into its third and final energy option, aerobic respiration. Glucose and free fatty acids are the primary fuels used during aerobic respiration.

What does all this have to do with getting the most from your workouts? Everything. Aerobic and anaerobic exercise affects your body in different ways. Both play an important role in becoming fit, regardless of your individual fitness goals. Excluding one of them from your exercise program means you are not taking advantage of your body's full potential; hence maximal results are not possible. To fully understand this concept, you need to know the pros and cons of aerobic and anaerobic exercise to see how they work together for maximum results.

We'll start with aerobic exercise. Aerobic exercise causes several things to occur in the body: heart rate accelerates, breathing increases, blood pressure rises. Now, all of this happens for a very good reason - to get oxygen (and nutrient) rich blood to your working muscles. Why should you care about oxygen? If oxygen is present, the body can use fat as fuel. Therefore, exercises that use the aerobic system burn fat.

But wait, there's more. Aerobic exercise performed in a progressive manner on a regular basis will make your muscles more efficient at processing fat. As your aerobic fitness improves, several cellular changes occur within the muscles. Mitochondria, sausage-shaped structures present in muscle cells, create ATP and metabolize fat. Keep getting aerobically fit and your mitochondria will multiply. Enzymes that break down fat will increase. These two changes will encourage muscles to take up more fat and use it. This is a good thing!

Fat burning aside, cardiovascular exercise offers many other benefits. Aerobic exercise burns calories, which is essential for weight management. It strengthens the heart and lungs so that they perform more efficiently. It reduces the chance of a heart attack or stroke. Endurance and energy levels increase. Blood circulation is enhanced. And, aerobic exercise positively impacts stress, anxiety, and depression. Be sure to read Champion Jason T. Hoffman's chapter where he explores 'The Other Benefits of Exercise.'

Wow, it sounds like aerobic exercise does it all. But wait - don't put on those running shoes yet. Aerobic exercise has a dark side. First, it does very little to stimulate muscle growth. Second, cardiovascular exercise does not improve your resting metabolic rate. Third, aerobic exercise done at too high an intensity or for too long can actually decrease fat usage and sometimes break down muscle tissue.

So what's the big deal about muscle anyway? Recall that anaerobic means "without oxygen." Building muscle is an anaerobic process. Remember those mitochondria, the ATP powerhouses that break down fat and use it for energy? Where are those little guys located? You got it…in muscle! Fat is burned in your muscles. The more muscle you have, the more efficient your body will be at using fat as a fuel source.

It gets better. Our bodies constantly need energy. Energy to think, breathe, move, and talk. The process of using calories for energy is commonly referred to as metabolism. As Champion Dan Houston notes in his chapter, 'Understanding Metabolism,' there are three ways your body uses calories - resting metabolic rate (RMR), physical activity and digestion, or the thermic effect of food. I know it's been mentioned by my fellow Champions but I think it bears repeating - muscle is metabolically active, fat is not. It requires energy (calories) to survive. Increasing your muscle mass means, get this…you will burn more calories while you sleep, sit, and hang out!

The second element of metabolism is physical activity. The activities you perform throughout the day require calories. One pound of fat is equal to 3,500 calories. To lose one pound of fat requires creating an energy deficit of 3,500 calories. Exercise is the best way to do that. Doing anaerobic and aerobic exercise burns calories that can lead to fat loss. And, the more muscle you have, the more calories you will expend while exercising.

Digestion is the third component that makes up your metabolism. The process of breaking down nutrients into their usable form, known as the thermic effect of food, requires a lot of energy. Champion Kelly Huggins' chapter, 'Burn Fat by Eating More!,' provides the details of the thermic effect of food that will convince you of this important element in utilizing food for energy.

Anaerobic exercise has even more to offer than just elevating your RMR and calorie burning to facilitate fat loss. Resistance training makes your bones stronger, helping to keep osteoporosis at bay. Strong muscles contribute to preventing injury by acting as shock absorbers, minimizing stress to the bones and joints. Further, let's not forget that anaerobic exercise can also reduce high blood pressure, improve your cholesterol profile, and enhance glucose metabolism.

Anaerobic exercise has one major flaw. It doesn't adequately challenge your cardiovascular system. And since you've read this far, you know how important the heart and lungs are to be healthy and to lose fat.

Is it crystal clear why you need to do both aerobic and anaerobic exercise? Each one provides benefits that the other cannot. Aerobic exercise strengthens your heart and lungs. It burns calories and fat. Anaerobic exercise builds essential muscle so that fat can be processed as a fuel. It boosts your metabolism at rest and while exercising.

Only when you combine the two can your fitness desires be achieved. Think of aerobic and anaerobic exercise as the offense and defense of a football team. Separately, they can stand on their own. But working together, they can develop into a championship caliber team that will go all the way to the Super Bowl.

So what will you do with your body? Will you take advantage of the benefits aerobic and anaerobic exercise has to offer? Or will you allow your fitness success to get sidelined?

Heath Gay, B.S., ACE

719-651-7497
Heath.Gay@thepowerofchampions.com
www.rockymountainfitnessservices.com

Always Finding a New Stimulus by Clint Phillips

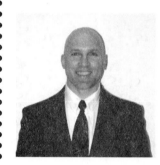

Champion Clint Phillips of Chicago, Illinois is one of the area's top personal trainers. He has trained everyone from Ironman triathletes to 600 pound teenagers and people in wheelchairs. Clint believes that fitness should be fun.

Did you ever see the movie 'Groundhog Day?'

In it, Bill Murray plays a weatherman who falls into a time warp in which he keeps reliving the same day over and over again. Before long, he is so frustrated and bored that he tries to kill himself by driving his truck off a cliff.

Unfortunately, many people conduct their exercise programs the same way. They keep repeating the exact same workout, day after day, week after week, until they are so jaded that they decide to put a stop to the whole thing.

Always doing the same workout is one of the biggest mistakes you can make, for three important reasons:

1. It quickly becomes boring; you'll soon hate your "routine."

2. It causes repetitive stress injuries because you always stress the same tendons and joints, from the same angles.

3. It is ineffective. Your body quickly adapts to the stimulus, and no longer needs to change or improve to keep up.

I've worked in the same fitness center for over five years, and have gotten acquainted with many of our regular patrons. Some come in to work out five times a week, for an hour each time - and they still look the same today as they did five years ago. What a colossal waste of time! They could mix up their routines a bit, spend half as much time exercising, and get better results. They'd also enjoy it more, and suffer fewer injuries.

Here are some great ways to vary your exercise program:

Vary the Number of Repetitions: I'm often asked, "How many reps should I do?" People want a magic number that will get them in great shape quickly. There is no magic number. The best way to workout is to vary the number of reps. Some days, do a high-rep workout, perhaps twelve to fifteen reps of each exercise. Next time, do a low-rep workout, maybe five or six reps of each. Another time, mix it up by doing one high-rep set, one medium-rep set, and one low-rep set.

Vary the Weight: How much weight should you lift? Lift enough weight to induce momentary muscle failure at the number of reps you've chosen. If you do a set of ten reps, number ten should exhaust you. If you can do eleven, twelve, or thirteen reps, pick a heavier weight next time. If you can get only five reps, try less weight next time. The weight and the number of reps always go together this way. To do a set of ten reps, pick a lighter weight than if you were going to do six.

Vary the Number of Sets: Beginners should start out by doing one hard set for each muscle group, then evaluate the results. If they are really sore, they should keep it at one set until they can handle more. After they've been working out for a while, most people can do three or four sets for each muscle group. But vary this too. If you are doing a light, very high-rep set, one may be enough. I recently had a client do 500 bodyweight squats. After that one set, his legs didn't need any more exercise for a few days! On the other hand, if you are doing very low-rep sets, do five or six sets. Doing more than six sets for any muscle group is usually overtraining and can do more harm than good.

Change the Exercises: This is where it gets fun! You can choose from literally thousands of exercises, so why do the same ten or twelve exercises repeatedly? If you workout with machines, try free weights. If you workout with dumbbells, try bodyweight calisthenics. Try adding some medicine ball drills. You can get a complete workout using nothing but a Swiss Ball. Tired of running on the treadmill? Try walking instead, but crank up the elevation. If you usually use the exercise bike, throw in a workout on the elliptical trainer, or try an aerobics class. Most fitness centers have at least ten different kinds of aerobics classes. Try them. Here are some things I've had my clients do, just to keep it fun and interesting:

- Boxing drills—Hit a heavy bag or focus mitts.
- Climb real stairs—If you live in a city with tall buildings, find the tallest one and climb the stairwell. Take the elevator down; climb it again.
- Wear a weight vest while doing your entire workout.
- Duplicate standard weightlifting exercises using rubber tubing instead of weights.
- Workout with a Body Blade.
- Use foam roller exercises.
- Use a Bosu.
- Borrow exercises from yoga or Pilates.
- Do balance work.
- Try partner exercises using manual resistance.

The Outer Edge—for serious exercisers who are ready for a challenge:

- Lift odd objects: sandbags, rocks, logs.
- Plyometric drills.
- Obstacle courses.
- Lift Kettle Bells.
- Swing Indian Clubs.
- Run laps in the shallow end of a pool.
- Push my car for laps around an empty parking lot while I steer from inside (my favorite).

Change the Speed of Movement: Standard weightlifting is done at a moderate pace. Olympic lifting is done quickly and explosively. Some trainers like the Super Slow style - one repetition takes anywhere from ten seconds to a full minute! I recommend standard weight lifting about 70-80% of the time, but throw in a Super Slow or Olympic workout occasionally.

Change the Range of Motion: Some say that every exercise should always be done through its full range of motion. Not true! Strength gains come three ways: more weight, more reps, and fuller range-of-motion. Most power lifters do a "three board press." At first, they may not be able to lift 300 pounds for five reps. If they stack three boards on their chest, and bring the weight down to touch the boards (not the chest) before pressing it up, they can get five reps. In a few weeks, they remove one board, and try for five reps. A few weeks later, they remove another board. Soon they are able to lower the weight all the way to the chest. Even if you don't want to become a power lifter you can steal some of their techniques.

Vary the Amount of Rest: Most people spend too much time resting. After a hard set, they do nothing for a minute or two. A better alternative is to immediately begin a new set that uses different muscles. After a set of biceps curls, do a set of lunges or crunches. While resting your arms, work the legs or abs.

Change the Order of Exercises: If you love structure, and want to keep the same routine for a couple of weeks, introduce variety by changing the order of your exercises. Say that your workout has fourteen exercises. Simply, label them "A" through "N." The first time, start with exercise A, and continue in order through exercise N. Next time, start with B, continue through N, and then do A. Start the third workout with C, continue through N, then do A and B.

Varying your exercise program is extremely important, but don't do it haphazardly. A good personal trainer can help you vary your routine in a scientifically orchestrated manner. But make sure you are getting your money's worth! I see a lot of people working out with personal trainers. Usually the trainer is reading from a clipboard, saying something like, "Okay, now we'll do curls with twelve-pound dumbbells, fifteen reps. Ready? One . . . two . . . three. . . ." That is not personal training. These people are professional clipboard-holders. They are professional rep-counters. They should hand the clipboard to the client and go sit down. Insist on getting what you pay for. All of my clients can count to fifteen without help. They depend on me to give them a great workout. That means they never do the same workout twice.

You don't wear the same clothes every day. You don't eat the same meal or watch the same TV show every day. Don't settle for the same workout again and again. You'll get much better results when you realize that the best routine is not to have a "routine" at all.

Clint Phillips, CSCS*D, ACE, AFAA

Clint.Phillips@thepowerofchampions.com
www.clintphillips.com
www.notimetoexercise.com

Ab-solute Truth: Sit Ups Won't Do It! by Todd Scott

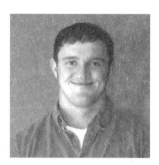

Champion Todd Scott of Baton Rouge, Louisiana is the owner of an elite personal training studio, Results! Fitness. His unlimited creative ability guides his clients to fitness success. You can obtain his free report, "17 Ways to Slash Fat Off Your Midsection," on his website.

"If you think you can, you can.

And if you think you can't, you're right!" Mary Kay Ash, Mary Kay Cosmetics

Many times in the gym I overhear members talking with one another or with the local gurus: 'I've got a big party coming up,' 'Summer's almost here,' or 'I just want to get rid of my beer belly.' Then they ask, 'What are the best exercises to flatten my stomach?'

And just as often the response goes something like this: 'Well, you should do 15 sets of butterfly crunches followed by 10 sets of oblique hammers and top it off with a few side bends.'

This is one of the places the confusion begins. Gurus "in the know" spread the myth that doing sit ups alone will actually burn the fat off your 'stomach' and create washboard abs. I'd like to clear up one thing first - stomach is not a synonym for abdominals. The abdominals are muscles that help to stabilize your body while the stomach is where food is digested.

Many people fall victim to misinformation spread by gym 'gurus,' letters, ads, marketing material, and content printed in health and fitness magazines that promise six-pack abs in 30 days, watch TV and burn the pounds, trap your fat and make it disappear, or electro-force your way to a flat tummy, 2 minutes a day, 3 days a week. These new ab routines aren't necessarily the key to a flat midsection . . .

And 2 minutes a day just ain't enough!

Well let's get to it . . .

What's the secret to slash fat off your waist? Reverse Crunch? Regular Crunch? Incline Sit Up? Bicycle Crunch? Hanging Leg Raise? V-Sit Up?

Hold on just a second!

I'm here to tell you that there is no pill, secret exercise, or magic gadget for what you're looking to achieve. But you have come to the right place, my friend.

Let's listen in on a recent conversation that I had with a frustrated fitness enthusiast:

Jane: Todd, I've been doing this new ab exercise for 2 months. At first it seemed like my waist was shrinking but now I think it may be getting bigger!

Me: Really? That's actually not too uncommon. What's the new ab exercise called?

Jane: It's called the Reverse Frog Crunch! It's a really neat exercise that I read about in the latest health magazine. I can really feel the burn!

Me: Wow! Can you show me how to do it?

As Jane moves into a position you'd only see in a game of Twister, her face begins to turn red as she counts backwards from 10!

Jane: (now grunting) I can only do a few of these because they really burn.

Me: Yeah, I can understand how you can only do a few, it looks like it really hurts. So you're telling me that you've been doing this for 2 months and haven't seen any results?

Jane: Yep. They promised a flat tummy in 8 weeks. I'm confused. Am I doing this wrong? I just have a few inches that I want to get rid of around my waistline and I figured that if I do these Reverse Frog Crunches it'll be gone no time. Is there any other abdominal exercise that will work better so I can lose fat?

Sadly, Jane is not alone in her quest for perfect abs in 60 days. These "information sources" work to either steal your money, keep you purchasing their products, or to just spread their ignorance. They want you to think that it's like waking up every morning to brush your teeth, just a routine! And they do this by conveniently forgetting to tell you about the three key components to having the tummy you've always wanted:

1. Supportive Nutrition - A balanced meal plan consisting of a lean protein, a starchy carbohydrate, and a fibrous carbohydrate consumed 5 - 6 times per day, 3 - 3.5 hours apart.

2. Moderate Aerobic Exercise - Aerobic exercise that increases your heart rate into your Target Heart Zone (THZ) and maintained consistently for a minimum amount of time.

3. A Concern for Muscle - Incorporating resistance exercise to maintain or increase muscle mass.

What? You're kidding me? You mean I can't do the super-duper upside down spider crunch and get a flat belly? Nope.

Let's briefly go over the anatomy of the abdominal muscles before we really dig in to distinguish between the truth and what's really just filling up space.

The abdominals are composed of several muscles: the Rectus Abdominus, Transverse Abdominus, and the External and Internal Obliques.

The abdominal muscles sit on the front and sides of the lower half of the torso, originating along the rib cage and attaching along the pelvis.

Functions

Rectus Abdominus - Flexes the spine (bringing the rib cage closer to the pelvis). This is seen in the abdominal crunching movement.

Transverse Abdominus - Acts as a natural weight belt, keeping your insides in. This muscle is essential for trunk stability.

Internal and External Obliques - Work to rotate the torso and stabilize the abdomen.

First of all, understand this: abs are muscles, there is no such thing as spot reduction (exercising a particular problem area to burn overlying fat, i.e., sit ups to burn abdominal fat), and without the three key components listed above, no abdominal routine will get you what you want. Period.

Your abdominals work together to provide stability, flexion, and rotation. The exercises are designed to stimulate your muscles to grow and to tone them up (the hardness of a muscle in a relaxed state; not the measure of fat on top of the muscle). That's it.

Have you ever done the "latest innovative ab routine" to burn fat off your belly? If you have, did it work? If you're reading this, it probably didn't. And if it appeared to, then it was only perceived fat loss.

Once you had 'toned' the muscles underneath the fat, your waistline appeared to be smaller and firmer. Since the muscle was toned (the hardness of a muscle in a relaxed state) and more compact, the overlying fat was drawn in. It was a mirage. And these 'results' can be seen in a matter of days. That's why companies guarantee you will lose inches not fat!

So, the new exercise routines and exercise machines that claim a 1" or 2" reduction in your waistline are not completely bogus. The fact is when you tone the muscle underneath the fat you can appear smaller. But the fat is still there!

Here's how the three components work together to create a lean waistline:

1. **Supportive Nutrition** - Eating smaller meals throughout the day helps keep insulin levels consistent, which is an important factor to burn fat. It also helps speed metabolism and deters fat

storage. When you eat frequent small meals that are consumed only for immediate energy requirements, there will be no excess calories to be stored as fat.

2. **Moderate Aerobic Exercise** - Aerobic exercise performed in your THZ efficiently burns fat by minimizing glycogen use and increasing the release of fat for fuel. Champion Heath Gay details the benefits of aerobic activity and fat loss in his chapter, 'The Two A's of Exercise Success.'

3. **A Concern for Muscle** - Since muscle is where fat is burned, it is important that it is maintained, if not increased. Each pound of muscle burns approximately 35-50 calories per day. Imagine if you lost 5-10 pounds of muscle what that would do to your metabolism! You guessed it. Fat-burning potential would be severely reduced! You may 'get' smaller but you will only be a smaller version of your old self. Reading Champion Peter Piranio's chapter, 'A Concern for Muscle,' will further convince you of the importance of the fat-burning potential of strength training.

Honestly, you can do ab exercises until you are blue in the face. If you aren't implementing the three key components (Supportive Nutrition, Moderate Aerobic Exercise, and A Concern for Muscle) it is possible to look and feel worse than when you started! Huh?

Here's the deal. When you begin an ab routine without these key components, your abs grow underneath the fat ultimately 'pushing' your fat outward and making your waist look bigger! By doing this, you can make yourself look worse!

Is that what you want?

If your goal is to obtain a six pack or a flat tummy, I'm not saying ignore abdominal work. In fact, for the best appearance of your abdominal muscles, it's imperative that your abs get developed. Just be sure that you are implementing supportive nutrition and moderate aerobic exercise and have a concern for muscle before you decide to get that perfect midsection.

Todd Scott, ACE, ISSA

7520 Perkins Suite 320
Baton Rouge, La 70808
(225) 241-6967
Todd.Scott@thepowerofchampions.com
www.toddscottfitness.com

Strength Training for Life by Mark Cibrario

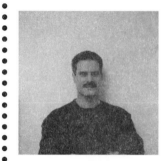

Champion Mark Cibrario of Waukegan, Illinois is the owner of The Trainers Club and serves as a consultant for Spri and Harbinger. He has produced 13 videos on strength training and authored books for Spri. His latest CDs include 'Functional Integrated Multi-Plane Stretching' and 'Functional Strength and Movement Assessment.'

As we age, do our bodies have to become increasingly less efficient in their ability to perform activities of daily living, manual labor/work tasks, or athletic movement?

If we observe the movement capabilities of most Americans, we would come to the conclusion that we're losing the battle. As 50 years of age is reached, or sadly even earlier, simple tasks such as dressing, rising up out of a chair or car seat, walking up and down stairs, or walking briskly are very challenging for many. Gardening, standard household activities, and light lifting tasks oftentimes have to be avoided. Participation in team or individual sports, personal recreational activities, and playing athletic games with children or grandchildren becomes increasingly more challenging.

With the exception of a functional debilitating orthopedic injury or physical handicap, we can maintain a high level of functional movement throughout our lives. One of the keys to victory is performing regular resistance training or weight training with the intent of improving our functional capabilities.

There are many strength training methods available to the consumer, which has created a lot of confusion as to what form may be the most beneficial for our bodies. Is the best method found at a Pilates studio, Super Slow training center, Curves center, or performing a machine circuit at a local health club? Can the best method be found through home training products such as the Bow Flex or Total Gym? Could it come from good old-fashioned strength training? This refers to using your own body weight, medicine balls, dumbbells, a barbell, and resistance training with the addition of modern cable pulley systems or rubberized resistance. If you guessed the last one, you're right!

I'm sure you've heard the saying, "If your goal is to run faster, practice running faster." Notice they didn't say ride a bike or swim more often. In this same context, if you want your body to become a more efficient mover when you are functioning in life, you should move in a life-like manner when training with resistance. To quote the father of functional rehabilitation, Gary Gray, "You can't learn to dance while sitting on your pants."

The key factor that separates all forms of resistance training comes down to 'function.' The important point to ponder is - does the involved method improve your ability to enhance your function within the environment in which you live and the activities you desire to participate in? This question applies whether you are a teenager or a senior citizen. To take full advantage of and maintain your body's God-given movement abilities, you should regularly perform what is referred to as essential movement pattern weight training with the good old-fashioned tools mentioned above. The primary movements include: balancing, pushing, pulling, reaching, carrying, lifting, lunging, squatting, stepping up/down, bending, extending, and auxiliary movements such as rotating, pivoting, and shifting. In addition, beyond the essential movement patterns, other conditioning exercises should be added depending on your activity profile such as: walking, jogging, sprinting, hopping, skipping, multi-directional agility drills, and jumping.

As we function in a life-like manner, all human movement emanates from the essential movement patterns. They are usually mixed and matched in many different combinations depending on the movement task. A very important point regarding improving function is that patterns are performed primarily while on your feet versus being in a seated or lying position. While standing, the stance or trunk angle can be altered to create a myriad of options to match the profile of human movement. You can select a square stance (wide, moderate, or narrow), split stance, single leg stance, or in some cases, a fencer's stance. You are also free to step, lunge, shift, or pivot in any direction. The trunk can hinge, bend, extend, laterally flex, and rotate freely. The key is that our trunk, hips, thighs, and buttocks are free to dynamically move in any direction or assume a stationary position to provide a solid platform for the upper extremities to work. It is very important that your hips, thighs, and buttocks are incorporated during functional movement as they serve to protect your back and spine by sharing the load and buffering forces imposed upon the spine.

When strength training is performed utilizing real life stances and trunk angles, the body's core, (thighs, hips, abdominals, obliques, low back musculature, and encompassing deep corset musculature) has to work together as a unit with the rest of the body. Your core is used as a connector for the lower and upper extremities and allows the body to function as one comprehensive core-generated unit. It is important to understand that if you are trying to improve your overall functional capabilities, you should not provide support systems under the buttocks or against the spine. When sitting or lying down, you are attempting to isolate muscular regions while disassociating the rest of the body. Traditional weight training and bodybuilding have taught us this method, but it is easy to see that we have been deceived.

Additionally, it is important to create bodily reactions that make you maintain and continually regain your center of gravity over your base of support, which prevents you from falling or stumbling. Performing resistance training in this real life three-dimensional gravity reactive environment, while speeding up your reflex responses, is critical to maintaining a healthy movement system and reducing the chance of injury. Also, training in this manner increases the body's ability to awaken and activate dormant stabilizing muscles, especially around critical joints such as the spine, shoulder, pelvis, hips, knees, and feet. Hiring an experienced trainer who has received continuing education in the areas of ideal postural alignment, flexibility screening, motor control, and functional movement coaching is a wise investment when learning to implement a functional training program.

Remember that your goal is to perform life-like essential movement pattern weight training, not to isolate parts of the body in foreign positions that you most likely never find yourself in. If you lie on the floor or use a machine that supports your body in any way (seated, prone [on your stomach], supine [on your back], or side lying), you are not teaching your body to be prepared for life's movement demands. The further you deviate from life-like movement patterns, especially when sitting and lying down, the less likely the exercise is to be beneficial to enhancing your human movement system and the more likely you are to incur injury. For this reason, I am not a proponent of seated or lying strength training unless rehabilitating from injury or attempting to add muscular hypertrophy.

In review, you should perform a large majority of strength training exercises within the scope of the essential movement patterns. They should be performed primarily in a standing position and next in other gravity-resisted positions (bent over, push up, kneeling) to create activation of the core musculature, which links the upper and lower extremities. Exercises should create a total body challenge to your body and heighten your awareness of reflexive balance and ideal posture from the head/neck down to the toes. Remember to move your body in a multi-directional or multi-plane manner, and not train like a robot.

Upper body exercises should incorporate static or dynamic participation from the lower extremities such as partial squatting and lunging prior to pushing and pulling as well as progressively incorporating dynamic hip and trunk shifting, rotating, and pivoting. Two arm actions are very traditional and still very useful, but one arm cable, tubing and dumbbell exercises should be a large part of a functional program as they allow us to perform patterns in several planes of movement. Lower extremity training should focus on single leg variations of the step-up, lunge, squat, Romanian dead lift, and cable-resisted hip focused patterns. Again, train in several planes of movement with these exercises to complement traditional two leg exercises.

Lastly, regarding the core, remember that the musculature is engaged during all essential movement pattern training. If you want to target core recruitment and improve your function, allow the hip complex and upper extremities to move freely in space. Your trunk muscles are activated best when stabilizing or holding the trunk rigid, or combining flexing and extending, laterally flexing, and rotating.

If you adhere to these guidelines, you will significantly increase your functional strength and health of the working joints, motor skills, and problem-solving skills as you encounter life's movement challenges. You will also greatly reduce the chance of incurring an orthopedic injury. Additionally, you will improve your posture, increase lean muscle mass and bone density, increase energy output or caloric expenditure, and have much more fun.

Mark Cibrario, CSCS/CPT NSCA, ACE

The Trainers Club Inc.
640 Anthony Trail
Northbrook, IL 60062
847-562-1611
Mark.Cibrario@thepowerofchampions.com

Functional Training: Breaking the Bonds of Traditionalism by Juan Carlos Santana

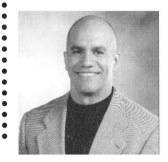

Champion Juan Carlos Santana of Boca Raton, Florida, a renowned authority on training and conditioning, is the director of the Institute of Human Performance. Juan Carlos serves as a consultant to major equipment manufacturers, sports teams, and fitness organizations.

For the last four decades, the bodybuilding approach to fitness has dominated the way we all strength train with weights.

Regardless of whether you want to play better tennis, look better, or rehab an injury, three sets of 10-15 reps on all the machines was the prescription of choice. "Bodybuilding for all" has been the predominant weight training theme in gyms for the last half century. Go to any gym and ask a personal trainer to make your goals a reality. Regardless of the goal, you will end up counting between 10-15 reps on various machines. The results of this approach have been mixed. As far as putting on muscle, no problem, bodybuilding training will do the job. However, when it comes to "putting some hustle behind the muscle," the outcome may surprise you.

The claims that weight training would make the body inflexible, slow, and generally "muscle bound" have been labeled as myths. This is one of the reasons various athletes, such a pitchers, soccer players, boxers, golfers, tennis players, and others, have traditionally stayed away from weight training. Following suit, many exercise aficionados have chosen the cardio route to training in order to avoid the muscle-bound syndrome. Although these assumptions may not be well founded in science, the weight training myths are not completely without some truth.

In general, weight training can't be blamed for all the unwanted qualities its reputation has bestowed upon it. However, the type of weight training performed can have a profound effect on performance. The bodybuilding approach that has permeated the weight training and fitness culture concentrates on isolating muscles in order to provide a superior growth stimulus. The isolation of muscle is an effective approach for muscle growth, but leaves little to be desired in terms of enhancing coordinated movement. It is this major weakness that has earned bodybuilding its muscle-bounding reputation. Whether bodybuilding deserves this reputation or not is a philosophical question that is beyond the scope of this discussion. What is very much the focus of our discussion is to provide an alternative to weight training. A new method of physical training that is capable of creating the body everyone desires, both in terms of looks and function.

The last decade has seen a resurgence of a more holistic approach to physical conditioning; it has been coined "Functional Training" (FT). Functional Training is not a new concept; it has been around since the beginning of time. The main distinction between FT and bodybuilding training is that FT trains movements, not isolated muscles. Functional Training works on the concept of "specificity." The concept of "specificity" dictates that you get what you train for: if you train complex movements, you get better at moving; if you train one muscle, that muscle gets bigger. In simple terms, if you want to get better and stronger at an activity, you would instinctively rehearse the activity, or at least parts of that activity. In sports we always say the best training for a particular sport is that sport! Although this is an oversimplification of the concept of FT, it is its essence. Let's take a look at a more detailed example of how FT works.

If you went into any gym and told a trainer that you needed to improve your running ability, they would naturally strengthen your leg muscles using leg extensions, leg curls and leg presses. However, do you really kick your leg out, curl it in, or kick up while on your back when you run? Of course not! What are the movements you really need to improve? Let's start with some basic observations of running.

Running occurs one leg at a time. This means only one leg is in contact with the ground at a time. Second, when you run, your trunk rotates. This means that in order for your body to efficiently move forward, the upper and lower limbs must rotate in opposition. The rotation between your hips and shoulders cancels upper and lower body rotational forces and keeps you facing and moving forward in an efficient manner, just like balancing your tires and having proper alignment makes your car run more efficiently. In order for the trunk to have this rotational control of the shoulders and hips, it must be strong and stable. Now, how effective do you think the leg presses, leg curls, and leg extensions will be at improving your running ability? Not very! None of these exercises really match the "function" of running.

A more functional approach to train the running motion would include all of these very basic observations and incorporate them into the training program. This means that the basic observations describe functional exercises. For example, realizing that running occurs one leg at a time, a more functional exercise for "running strength" would be a single leg forward reach or single leg squat. Since one needs a very strong and stable core to control the rotation between the hips and shoulders, a more functional exercise for running would also be a medicine ball rotation. An unlimited version of these exercises allows the fitness professional to exactly match the intensity of the exercise with the fitness level of the client, making this approach to training not only effective, but more importantly, very safe!

Now, I know what you're thinking, "All of this sounds so logical it is hard to argue against." It is common sense, right? One would think so, but the problem with common sense is - it's not so common. One look in any gym and you will see 99 percent of the people training in a non-functional manner. In fact, many gyms spend as much as 75-95% of their equipment investment on non-functional equipment. Next time you go into your gym, check out how many people are doing machine leg extensions, machine leg curls, machine seated calf raises, machine rows, machine presses, machine everything! These pieces of resistance-training equipment are the most popular in most gyms, and the gauge by which many people evaluate the "productive worth" of training facilities. To the uneducated consumer, "the more machines the better!"

Tradition is hard to break. However, this tradition is slowly giving way to changes due to the influence of FT. We are starting to see more floor space, equipment, and group classes dedicated to more functional approaches to training.

Functional Training also has enormous impact on muscle quality, weight reduction and rehabilitation. Just look at gymnasts – are they not muscular and lean? Gymnasts have bodies most of our clients would die for: muscular, symmetrical and lean. Yet, they never lift weights or perform bodybuilding exercises. Gymnasts get their bodies through a FT approach: training movement not muscles. Since FT trains movements, it works many muscles at a given time. Because of this the caloric burn of FT is far superior to that of isolated bodybuilding exercises. The cardiovascular benefits of FT are also head and shoulders above bodybuilding, especially if done in a circuit-style format. Finally, the integration of multiple muscle systems enhances muscular balance and coordination. This has enormous implications in rehabilitation. A functional approach to rehabilitation has been shown to cut rehabilitation time by as much a 50%. I personally rehabilitated an ACL reconstruction in 9 weeks, usually a 6-month rehab time.

Functional Training has been slowly coming to the forefront of the fitness industry. Many personal trainers are embracing it because of its safe, effective and fun approach to developing human performance and enhancing physical aesthetics. This training approach has a deep and rich history that is surely repeating itself before our very eyes. So, keep your eyes and minds open to the future of fitness – Functional Training.

Juan Carlos Santana, M.Ed., CSCS

Institute of Human Performance
1950 NW 2nd Avenue
Boca Raton, Florida, 33432
561-620-9556
JC.Santana@thepowerofchampions.com
www.ihpfit.com
www.opsfit.com/carlos.html

Finding the Athlete Inside by David Thomas

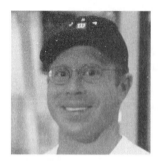

Champion David Thomas of Mountain Brook, Alabama is the founder and president of Total Fitness Consultants Inc., a personal training facility located in Birmingham, Alabama. David provides quality functional fitness programs for people from all walks of life.

Being a personal trainer/strength and conditioning coach has allowed me to work with a diverse group of clients.

Most clients have goals of losing body fat, strengthening their bodies, feeling better about themselves, and having a better quality of life. However, every so often that inspired client walks through my doors with dreams about reliving their childhood days when he or she scored the winning touchdown, hit the shot at the buzzer, or served the ace to win the match.

Many of these clients have stayed fairly active throughout their adult lives and have continued to participate in recreational or "weekend warrior" activities. Others come to me in despair about how their bodies have slowed as time has caught up to and passed by their youthful minds. When faced with the dilemma of how to train these Tiger Woods wanna be's, I meet each one with a solution that fits his or her lifestyle as well as their aspirations.

The first step in the program is to create tangible goals for what each individual wants to do and what he or she is currently able to do. An evaluation of current fitness and activity levels is a good indicator of the starting point when designing a strength and conditioning program.

Once this has been completed, we discuss how much time the person is willing to commit to a program. This indicates if they are serious about training or just trying to improve enough to beat their neighbor at a friendly golf match. Then we break it down based upon the specific sport and design a program that meets the demands of that sport and accommodates the current fitness level of the client. For example, a program for a client who has been sedentary for the past ten years but has goals of playing club soccer would be different from one prescribed for the client who has been weight training for ten years and then decides to hire me for an additional push or motivation.

When beginning a strength and conditioning program as a recreational athlete, you must first realize that this training program will and should be quite different from that of the training program you may be following to improve muscle tone and strength.

When designing programs for athletes, I look at several factors such as energy systems used, speed of movement, and planes of motions the body goes through during the sport. Muscle mechanics, recovery time, and external factors (balls, people, etc.) must also be addressed.

Energy Systems

Most athletes are aware that some sports require a higher and far different type of conditioning than other sports do. For instance, a football player's conditioning plan would be far different from that of a soccer player. A golfer would require far less cardiovascular training than a basketball player.

When deciding how to design a program, look at the energy systems used. Does your sport require a higher level of cardiovascular output (VO_2 max)? Does the sport require repetitive sprints for thirty yards and then recovery to a slow jog or even stop for a brief period, or is there a need for continuous cardiovascular output? This information is needed to determine how much or how little cardiovascular training is required in a program for optimal performance. The worst thing you can do when training for a particular sport is to train the wrong energy system. Imagine if a football player spent all of his time doing long distance runs for his workouts. You must train in the same manner as you play.

Speed of Movement

Speed of movement is a component of training that ties into the energy system. During the evaluation of the sport, look at how fast or slow and in what manner you are moving. Are most movements done in a slow methodical manner or are you moving at high speeds in place as well as over distance? Most people think of speed as distance covered over ground; however, a body can move extremely fast and stay in the same spot. Speed of movement has to be assessed in both ways.

Periodization

Periodization is a concept of training that is often talked about but frequently misunderstood by many novice exercisers. Simply put, periodization is designing your program into phases in conjunction with the time of year at which your sport is active. A good basic principle is to break the calendar year down into four components based upon your sport's off-season, pre-season, in-season, and post-season training period.

Periodization provides your body with the most effective volume and selection of exercises to achieve optimal performance. The key factors that determine a good periodization program are sets, reps, rest, intensity and percentage of a 1 RM (repetition max weight). The program must be designed with these factors in mind.

I have trained several athletes that had been doing the same exercises, sets, reps and rest throughout the entire year. By following the same routine, these individuals allowed their bodies to adapt to that routine. As a result, they did not get maximum benefits from their training, nor did their bodies grow or heal properly.

Overuse injuries often occur to people who do not monitor their training variables, and burnout often occurs for those who do not manipulate training variables. A good periodization program allows your body to get stronger and more conditioned in the off-season and to maintain these gains during the season. The primary goal of a strength program during the sport season is to maintain the strength and power already obtained and keep the nervous system firing at optimal performance levels; periodization can help an athlete accomplish these goals.

A complete program set up with changes in these training variables will allow your body to adapt and grow stronger. Champion Brian Schiff offers a more detailed exploration of this topic in his chapter, 'Periodization.'

Functional Strength Training

Recently, functional training has been receiving a tremendous amount of attention. Functional training means creating an exercise program that closely resembles movements of a specific sport. An athlete's needs in his sport must be addressed when designing a program. Moving from machine to machine counting out ten reps will not properly prepare the body for the demands of an athletic event.

Regardless of the sport or activity, an exercise program should contain movements specific to your sport. You should also incorporate exercises that will address any weaknesses you may have. This may include muscle weaknesses or imbalances, flexibility issues, chronic injuries, and any other problems that may interfere with the program selected.

The best way to design your sports program is to create an environment that does several things. Create or implement multi-dimensional patterns by training your body in all three planes of movement. Front to back (sagittal), side-to-side (frontal) and rotational (transverse) are all movement patterns required to ensure a balanced program.

Using a propriosensory (balance) component that challenges the body and brain to work together is essential in training an athlete. In sport, a person's body works as a complete unit, so it should be trained accordingly. This can and will add a degree of difficulty to the program. Free-weight exercises are well suited to achieve this. There is a higher learning curve to training with free weights, but once mastered, progression and advancement are almost automatic.

When clients who have been following the same training program for years are exposed to the benefit of training in this manner, they see rapid results. Within weeks, many of these clients are jumping higher, running faster, and redeveloping skills they once had as college athletes. I am convinced this component is critical for the success of the advanced or even the recreational athlete.

Champions Mark Cibrario and Juan Carlos Santana delve more deeply into the benefits of functional training in the two previous chapters.

Summary

Training for sports does require more planning than the basic workout. A properly planned exercise program that relates to a specific sport can be extremely beneficial to a recreational athlete. When designing your program, consider your current fitness level, the time you have to devote to training, and what your goals are. Having an organized plan allows you the freedom to train properly and efficiently, to exercise consistently, to reach your goals, and most of all, to have fun.

David Thomas, CSCS, ACE

11 Dexter Avenue, Mountain Brook, AL 35213
2833 Culver Road, Mountain Brook, AL 35223
205-871-7744
David.Thomas@thepowerofchampions.com

Adventure Racing Training for the Weekend Warrior by Matt McKinnis

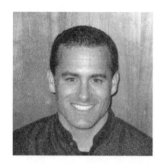

Champion Matt McKinnis of Alexandria, Virginia has been a cycling instructor/personal trainer for over 4 years. He is certified through Reebok Spinning, American Council on Exercise (ACE) and is CPR and First Aid certified through the American Red Cross.

The sport of adventure racing has been gaining popularity for the past ten years.

With the help of the most popular race, The Eco-Challenge, people all over the world want to know how they can train for their first adventure race. For most people the sport is very addictive so be prepared to be bitten by the adventure racing bug and join me at one of the races.

There are primary and secondary disciplines in adventure racing and it is essential to train for all of them. The primary disciplines, mountain biking, hiking, and paddling, are components of each adventure race. In addition, the Race Director will add secondary disciplines to make it more interesting and challenging. They can vary from getting your teammates over a 45 degree, 12 foot wall covered in Crisco to crawling through caves in several inches of muddy water on your hands and knees.

The good news is once the primaries have been mastered the secondary ones are easier to conquer. It is important to train based on the length of race, which includes 3 main categories: the sprint races which range from 3 to 6 hours; 24-, 36- and 48-hour races; and expedition races which range between 5 and 10 days.

The three elements to concentrate on are endurance training, weight training and nutrition. These three will properly prepare you to cross the finish line.

Mountain biking for me is one of the best overall disciplines. My first love is biking, both road and mountain, so I might be somewhat biased. The race directors create challenges for the biking courses, which are very unforgiving but truly exhilarating. The majority of the mountain biking sections are done on forest service roads with very little done on single-track courses, which means you do not need the proficiency demanded of single track. The sections are long and "hilly" and you must prepare your cardiovascular system and legs for this challenge. In conjunction with this outdoor training, you need to do lower body weight training to build the muscles, which are used to climb, speed, and descend. Try the following exercises to strengthen your legs: squat, leg press, walking lunge, good morning, and leg curl.

Start with 3 sets of 10 repetitions for each exercise, and after three weeks advance to 3 sets of 15 repetitions. Every three weeks thereafter, progress to a new set of repetitions at 12, 10, 8 and then back up to 15. The change in repetitions lends a variety to the workout and ensures you won't get bored with the routine. This also helps to improve endurance and strength in the muscles. This weight training plan remains the same in training for all of the disciplines. Weight training must be performed 2 to 3 times a week. It is ideal to work two of the exercises each day to ensure work of the quadriceps and hamstrings.

Increasing endurance on the bike is very important. Start from the basics if riding has not been part of your program. A spinning class is a great start, because it helps build endurance and speed, and it is a must to start logging miles on the bike. Plan a weekly time to take long 20 plus mile outdoor rides. If starting from scratch, begin with a 5 mile ride. Always wear a heart rate monitor and use a computer which should be mounted on your bike. It is extremely important to maintain your heart rate at your targeted zone, which varies depending on age. Be sure to read Champion Brett Pruitt's chapter, 'Putting Your Heart into Your Exercise Program,' to learn more about determining and maintaining target heart rate. The computer on the bike will help you to maintain a good cadence with your pedaling. Increase the length of rides each week until you reach 50 miles. Set a goal of using a bike trainer 1-1 ½ half hours 2 to 3 times a week.

Nutrition is very important while training because your caloric needs increase due to the excessive endurance and weight training. An increase in protein, fats and carbohydrates is needed to help maintain strength and endurance during training and aids in a faster recovery after workouts. This nutrition plan remains the same throughout training in all of the disciplines.

Hiking is "make or break" time in an adventure race because there are multiple hiking sections. If not prepared for this discipline, it is extremely difficult to finish the race. The feet are exposed to severe conditions brought on by climate, terrain, and use, which means preparing this part of the body is a critical element of training. Running, preferably outdoors, is the best way to physically prepare your feet but a treadmill is also appropriate. Begin with a mile and increase the distance by a half mile to a mile each week. Schedule time weekly to do long outdoor runs. It is important to coordinate the long run days with the long biking days by altering from one to the other to ensure training is accomplished for both. The goal for long runs is to peak between 10 and 15 miles.

The second critical training regiment for hiking is hiking outdoors on actual trails which have elevation gains and are technical. Another important element is the weight of the backpack. The first hike will be for one hour with water in the pack. The goal is to incrementally add weight to the pack to replicate the weight of the gear carried during the race. Simultaneously increase the length of the hikes until reaching a goal of 4 to 6 hours per hike. The ultimate weight of the pack will be between 30 and 50 pounds. The differential is a result of the type of race for which the training is being done.

Weight training also involves increasing the weight as the training progresses. It is critical to add shoulder exercises to prepare for carrying the pack. The best exercises for the shoulders are dumbbell press, rear raise, shrugs, dumbbell lateral raise and high pull rope.

Paddling is a major element in adventure racing. In the multi-day races, there are several different disciplines of paddling, which vary from flat water to white water kayaking. The amount of time spent behind the paddle during the race makes it critical to prepare correctly. It is essential to both learn the correct paddle stroke while also learning how to pace to ensure completion of the segment. Never count on an easy section in paddling, because Mother Nature always plays a major role in reversing the downwind to an upstream wind. Begin this training in a kayak while noting the length of the kayak, which affects its speed and maneuverability. The longer it is the straighter it tracks. The more volume a boat has the more buoyant it is. It features a stable hull for comfort and confidence, true tracking for easier straight line paddling and a large safety cockpit for easy access and exit. Beginner boats are usually high volume and longer with a rounded bottom compared to advanced boats. The first workout should be at least an hour. It is essential to drink plenty of water during the workout. Increase the workout by a half hour to an hour each session. The gradual increase in time will help prevent injuries to overused muscles and tendons. Don't grip the paddle too tightly, because a "too tight" grip causes tendonitis in the elbow.

I have personally followed this training routine and have seen a dramatic improvement from my first race four years ago to ones recently completed in 2003. My body recovers much faster with the increased weight training and I am much stronger during the races. If you have ever thought about participating in an adventure race, this program will help you get stronger, faster, motivated and in the spirit. See you at the races!

Matt McKinnis, ACE

107 King Henry Court
Alexandria, VA 22314
703-898-7607
Matt.McKinnis@thepowerofchampions.com

Off-Set Training by Carter Hays

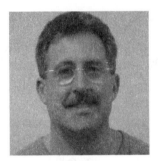

Champion Carter Hays of Houston, Texas has worked in the fitness field for over 25 years. He is currently a personal trainer, performance enhancement specialist, integrated flexibility specialist, and USAW Club-Coach.

Off-Set Training (OST) is a form of neuromuscular stabilization training (NST).

Two of the major goals of NST are enhancing static and dynamic balance while at the same time creating greater stabilization strength. OST is most effective in an integrated program, focusing on muscle systems and movement. OST can be performed in a single exercise format or with total body movement in a multi-planar proprioceptive rich environment. Because OST requires significant core (lumbo-pelvic-hip) stabilization skill, it is recommended for the intermediate or advanced trainee.

One of the major advantages of OST is the flexibility inherent in the method, and the freedom to use as many different training tools as possible. You can train indoors or outdoors, with dumbbells, medicine balls, powerballs, cables, tubing, bodyblades, kettlebells. You can also combine these different tools for greater challenges to stability and/or strength.

To generate better results and have more fun, you can utilize stability balls, benches, floor, steps, coreboards, grass, and hills. The combination moves you can create are endless; you can use double leg, single leg, squatting, lunging, step-ups, step-downs, step-overs, and so on. Like all training methods, to be successful with OST you must be physically prepared for this progression. You should be on an integrated flexibility program and have good core stability before undertaking the OST challenge.

For OST to enhance your training, you need to consider the benefits of the training in relation to your goals. Let's review some of the major benefits of OST:

OST challenges the core while performing static and dynamic exercises. The core is constantly trying to keep the back in a neutral posture during OST and creates significant stabilization strength and muscular endurance in the entire core musculature.

Because the stabilizers in the cervical/shoulder, lumbo-pelvic-hip, and knee/ankle regions become more stable and efficient, your prime movers, lats, pecs, delts, quads, and glutes, are more effective in their contractions (concentric, eccentric, and isometric), which can lead to better muscular development and performance. In addition, OST challenges the neuromuscular system. As a result, all muscles can act as stabilizers on occasion and ultimately help with injury–proofing your body.

OST is by nature a total body, multi-planar exercise format. It can be performed with double leg and single leg movements in short or longer sequences. This training method is a high intensity, high energy, demanding exercise that burns a significant amount of calories.

It is highly flexible and can be used as a couple of movements at the beginning of your regular workout or at the end of a workout prior to cool down. OST can also take the place of your current workout with single exercises and total body exercises done in horizontal sets. To challenge your cardiovascular system, it can be done in vertical sets.

OST helps create better mental acuity and physical coordination. Because you are typically moving with varying weights in each hand, i.e., combining movements like curls or presses with lunges or squats, you have to have excellent concentration skills. Your physical coordination will grow in leaps and bounds.

OST is meant to help you create optimal results and peak performance, not to stay at mediocre. Most importantly, OST is fun and challenging. If you add OST to your current training regimen, you will increase your results and minimize the chance of stagnation. It just might be the jolt your workout needs.

Now let's look at the way it's done.

Off-Set Training

For each exercise you will need to find a dumbbell (DB) that you can lift for 6-8 reps on one side and another that you can lift for 12-15 reps on the other side. Lock your core by drawing your belly button in toward the spine. During each exercise, be sure to move the dumbbells at the same speed and with equally efficient form. At the end of the first set, switch each dumbbell to the opposite hand for the next set.

For muscle systems, shoulders, chest, back, legs and total body exercises, perform the following exercises.

Dumbbell Shoulder Press. Press the weights shooting for a total of 8-12 reps.

Dumbbell Bench Press. Lie on the bench, make sure you are stable and press.

Dumbbell Bent Over Row. Maintain a solid neutral back throughout the exercise.

Dumbbell Lunge. You can do front lunges by keeping your hands on either side of your lunging leg. You can do alternating or same leg lunges, 45 degree lunges and backward lunges. Side lunges also work well. You will definitely feel the challenge to your core with these variations. Make sure to switch dumbbells for the next set.

Here's an example of a total body exercise using OST:

> <u>Alternating lunge/curl/press</u>, Grab a different weight DB in each hand as described above. Stand up straight with hands at your sides. Begin your lunge by stepping out with your right foot, as the right foot makes contact with the ground, begin your two arm curl, your right hand is on the outside of the right leg, your left hand is on the inside of the right leg. Your curl and full range of motion lunge should end at the same time. Your arms have completed the curl, your right leg is at 90 degrees and your left thigh is perpendicular to the floor. Your shoulders are over your hips and your core is tight. Now you perform a shoulder press with both hands. Keeping your back straight and core tight, push off with the right leg bringing your left foot back in line with your right. To really challenge the core, make sure your arms remain straight overhead in line with your ears. Once you have recovered, bring the DBs down to your shoulders and do a 4 count eccentric curl. Now you are in position to begin the next rep with your left side. Complete as described for your right side. Once you have completed a set of 8-12 reps, switch DBs to opposite hands.

This particular exercise is excellent at integrating the upper and lower body as well as right and left sides. Feel free to use DBs and power ball or any combination of resistance that works for you.

Exercise tips for building a great routine:

- Make sure that you can perform at least 6-8 reps with the heavy DB you choose. Your goal will be to eventually get to 15 reps with that weight. The greater the disparity in weight, the greater the challenge.

- Once you master any given movement, challenge yourself with different forms of resistance, alternating arms, single leg, or any combination that enhances your routine.

- If you are working with single off-set exercises, try going from a horizontal set format to a vertical set format for greater neuromuscular and cardiovascular challenge.

- Since OST is really a component of Neuromuscular Stabilization Training, it is best to keep your reps at 8-15 or higher and keep your pace moderate.

- You can also do different movements with different weight to challenge stabilization, <u>i.e.</u>, one hand is performing a shoulder press holding a 45 lb. DB while the other hand performs a lateral raise holding a 15 lb. DB. To challenge stabilization further, perform this movement on one leg, and switch for the next set.

OST is a training tool you can use to add dimension and challenge to your training program. It is not a be-all-and-end-all. If you desire an integrated, periodized program, OST can definitely move you closer to your goals.

Carter Hays, MC, NSCA-CPT, NASM-PES, NASM-IFS, USAW Club-Coach

281-924-3156
Carter.Hays@thepowerofchampions.com
www.carterhaystraining.com

The Routine that Worked Wonders by Stephen Holt

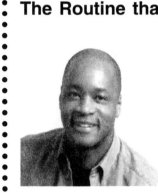

Champion Stephen Holt of Lutherville, Maryland was named The American Council on Exercise's Personal Trainer of the Year for 2003. He has helped literally thousands of exercisers over 20 years make their workouts both more productive and time-effective through his websites and workshops.

For over twenty years, I trained my clients the way everyone else did.

Then finally I started thinking for myself and discovered the Routine that Worked Wonders.

You see, the average program for the average person is based on bodybuilding lore – exercises that exist only because they have always existed. But one of the first things most of my clients say to me is, "I don't want to look like a bodybuilder." So why continue to train with exercises aimed at maximizing the size of a handful of individual muscles?

Your body has more than 600 muscles each connected to your bones in spiral and diagonal patterns, not in straight lines. Doesn't it make sense to acknowledge and respect these patterns in the exercises you do? Most traditional exercises, however, assume a straight-line connection, and many standard machines actually force you to move in straight lines.

Most of us aren't interested in living a bodybuilder's lifestyle. We don't have time to lift as long or as frequently as bodybuilders. We don't have time to do isolation exercises for every single muscle we can name – and even different heads of different muscles.

Think about it … how much time would you have to spend in the gym if you did an exercise for each head of the biceps, each head of the triceps, each head of the deltoids, each head of the quadriceps, etc.? No wonder you feel like you spend all day at the gym and still don't get much done.

The answer is to completely change the way you look at exercise. No more isolation movements that try to work one muscle head at a time.

The answer is to incorporate moves that work as many muscles as possible. Remember, the more muscle mass you use, the more calories you'll burn.

The answer is to work your muscles together the way they normally work everywhere but in the weight room.

My clients have reported outstanding fat loss, strength gains, and increased stamina using these techniques. More important, they have more fun, remain enthusiastic and just plain feel better – in addition to looking better.

The answer, and the Routine That Worked Wonders, is the 3-4-5 System:

- 3 Planes of Motion
- 4 Muscle Systems (not the "major muscle groups" that you've probably read about)
- 5 Fundamental Movement Patterns

Let's take a closer look at each of these.

3 Planes of Motion

The three planes of movement are the sagittal (front and back), frontal (side-to-side) and transverse (rotation).

The foundation of the "3" in the 3-4-5 System is that all muscles have some action in all three planes. So it makes sense to work in all three dimensions. Traditional bodybuilding exercises don't do that — not well, at least.

4 Muscle Systems

Here's where it gets a little complicated, but bear with me for a moment. You only need to understand the concepts for now, not the details. Recent research tells us certain muscles work together in four major groups or "systems" – don't be thrown by the fancy names though.

1. The Anterior Oblique System (AOS) connects your obliques and inner thigh muscles.

2. The Posterior Oblique System (POS) consists of your latissimus dorsi (lats) and gluteus maximus (glutes). The fibers of these two muscles are directly in line with each other. They also cross your sacroiliac (SI) joint and support this often-troublesome spot.

Since your glutes are the largest muscles in your body and your lats are the largest muscles in the upper body, working this system is excellent for calorie burning.

3. The Lateral System (LS) consists of the outer thigh and inner thigh muscles of one leg, and the opposite quadratus lumborum, a muscle often implicated in low back pain. These muscles act to keep you upright whenever you're on one leg (as in walking).

When you drive a car, for example, you're constantly steering slightly to the left and slightly to the right to keep the car moving in a relatively straight line. The same idea applies to your inner and outer thigh muscles. They work in unison to keep your hips relatively level and your knees facing relatively straight ahead as you move.

4. The Deep Longitudinal System (DLS) starts with a muscle connected to your big toe, goes up the side of your leg, and continues on to connect your hamstrings and the muscles along your spine. It's affected whenever your foot is on the ground and is a vital shock-absorption system.

To get the most of out of your LS and DLS, and to burn the most calories, you'll do most of your exercises standing.

5 Fundamental Movement Patterns

Now it gets simple, again. We break down movement into five general patterns: pulling, pushing, rotation, one leg stance and moving your center of gravity (COG).

Pulling exercises (moving your hands toward your body – like a row) help fortify your POS, and strengthen your mid-back, low back and the dozens of muscles along your spine.

Pushing exercises (moving your hands away from your body – like a chest press or shoulder press) integrate your chest, shoulder and arm muscles with your abdominals, while your hips and legs stabilize.

Pushing or pulling exercises using just one arm also accentuate the way your obliques, spinal and mid-back muscles all work together.

Rotation exercises emphasize your obliques and include the often-neglected rotational function of many other muscles including your hamstrings and inner thigh muscles.

Your hips should have a large degree of rotation, yet no machine strengthens this movement. More important, many people have lost the rotation in their hips and shoulder girdle, so when they rotate — as we do all day long – that rotation is focused in the spine. This can lead to low back pain.

Though they might appear harmful at first glance, standing rotational exercises can help restore hip and upper body rotation and actually decrease the stress on your low back.

One leg stance. Did you know that walking requires you to spend about 80 percent of your time on one leg or the other? Exercises that combine a one-leg stance with your foot hitting the ground (lunges are a prime example) teach your leg muscles to react subconsciously to keep you upright.

Moving your COG (as in a squat, for example) works virtually all of your lower body muscles in addition to your low back. COG exercises are great for teaching and reinforcing proper lifting mechanics and dynamic spinal stabilization.

Putting "3," "4" and "5" Together

Now you can combine the 3 planes of movement, 4 muscle systems and 5 fundamental movement patterns to make your workouts more efficient than ever before. It's not nearly as complicated as it seems at first.

Certain moves automatically fall into several groups at once. Any one leg exercise automatically works your Lateral System and at least one plane. Any one arm exercise for either the AOS or the POS will typically cover transverse plane and rotation.

Here's a sample 3-4-5 workout you can do using the cable cross unit available in most gyms:

Core (ab dominant)	Plank
Core (back dominant)	Bridge
Rotation	Reverse Woodchop
Pull	Cable One Arm Row
Push	Dumbbell One Arm Curl and Press
COG	Deadlift
One Leg	Dumbbell Side Lunge

It's really that simple. Keys are to:

- use your legs in each exercise
- use only one arm when possible
- incorporate rotation when possible

With my 3-4-5 System, you can work virtually all of your muscles in a single, time-effective session while increasing calorie burning during and after the workout, building at least a little more muscle (which is a good thing), alleviating boredom, and avoiding plateaus - all at the same time.

Knowing that you only have to cover three simple rules of all 3 planes, all 4 muscle systems and all 5 movement patterns ensures that you strengthen every muscle in a way that builds — not ignores — intermuscular coordination. At the same time, the flexibility of the "3-4-5 System" leaves much to your imagination and keeps your workouts fun, exciting and productive.

Give it a try and you'll never go back to your old routine.

Stephen Holt, BSE, CSCS, PES

410-453-6295
1-888-741-4900 toll free
Stephen.Holt@thepowerofchampions.com
http://345TotalBodyFitness.com
http://StephenHoltFitnessOnline.com

Periodization by Brian Schiff

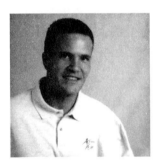

Champion Brian Schiff of Dublin, Ohio owns The Fitness Edge training studio. He is a licensed physical therapist with a background in sports medicine. He currently serves as a strength and conditioning specialist for The Columbus Crew Major League Soccer Team.

Do you ever wonder how to break out of a training rut or overcome plateaus in your workout?

Are you bored with your current exercise program? Do you question the manner in which you are training? Could you have better prepared for the most important competition to date? If you answered 'Yes' to any of these questions, then you share a similar problem with many who are constantly searching for the perfect training regimen. The human body is adept at adapting quickly to outside stimuli, therefore, it is imperative to carefully plan and manipulate certain variables within an exercise program to ensure maximal results. As such, the concept of periodization becomes critical in achieving your peak performance.

Periodization refers to a cyclical training strategy that is employed to avoid training plateaus, while preparing you for optimal performance at a certain point in time. Typically, a periodization plan is one year or longer, depending on the level of experience and skill of the individual, in addition to the time needed to reach the desired goal. This strategy is often used for athletes trying to peak for a competition. But, even if you are not a competitive athlete, please read on, as you will find these principles and techniques useful in traditional resistance training as well.

In this model of training, you manipulate volume, intensity, and specificity of exercise throughout planned periods or cycles. The annual plan is referred to as a macrocycle, which in turn consists of two or more mesocycles. The mesocycles last several weeks or months, and they consist of smaller, more specific training schedules known as microcycles. Due to the narrow focus of microcycles, they are typically adapted throughout the mesocycle based upon training progress and fatigue.

The concept of periodization was originally introduced in the 1960's by a Russian physiologist, Leo Matveyev.[18] It has since become more popular among many Western strength and conditioning professionals. Training intensity and volume are the two primary factors that are manipulated to attain the desired training effect. The training begins with an emphasis on higher volume low intensity exercise with little emphasis on sport-specific activity, and then shifts throughout the cycles to lower volume high intensity training with greater sport specificity as you lead up to the competitive event. More specifically, it is broken down into specific phases, known as preparatory, competitive and transition phases coinciding with the associated sports seasons.[19] In the conventional periodization model, the preparatory phase is followed by a first transition phase, prior to initiating the competitive phase.[20] However, upon completion of the competitive phase, standard periodization models also call for a transition phase (second transition in conventional model) consisting of unstructured active rest. This period typically lasts one to four weeks and consists of non-sport-specific activities designed to rejuvenate the central nervous system and allow the mind and body to rest prior to beginning a new training macrocycle.

The periodized training phases describe the specific manipulation of training variables. In the preparatory phase, you establish a base level of conditioning to prepare for future, more intense training. This phase is often the longest, and it is where most gains are accomplished. Within the preparatory phase, you can further divide the training into the hypertrophy phase, max (basic) strength phase and power phase.[19] This sequence of progressive training enables you to steadily raise intensity as you prepare for competition. It should also be noted that rest-to-work ratios for aerobic/anaerobic conditioning steadily decrease during the preparatory phase depending on the primary energy system trained and desired training effect. The phases are broken down as follows:

Hypertrophy Phase – The training load is 50-75% of 1 RM (repetition maximum), while utilizing 3-6 sets of 10-20 repetitions. This phase is designed to increase lean body mass and endurance. It provides a foundation to build strength and power in the later phases.

Max Strength Phase – The training load is 80-90% of 1 RM, while performing 3-5 sets of 4-8 repetitions. You now begin to perform more sport-specific strengthening and plyometric exercises. The goal of this phase is to maximize strength gains.

Power Phase – The training load is 75-95% of 1 RM, while further reducing volume to 3-5 sets of 2-5 repetitions. Even though the percent RM scale is lower at the bottom, you have to remember that many of the exercises are performed explosively and the relative intensity is higher. Additionally, you now perform more sport-specific drills and skills during this phase as competition draws near. For most athletes, training should focus on appropriate Olympic lifts, explosive movements and intense, specific plyometric training. The goal is to maximize power development, while continuing to increase strength.

After the preparatory phase concludes, you move into the competitive phase. The focus is on further reducing volume of training and increasing intensity to greater than 93% of 1 RM with 1-3 sets of 1-3 reps, if the desired effect is to continue working for greater gains. At this heightened intensity, it is only reasonable to peak for two to three weeks. However, over a long competitive season with multiple contests, your goal should be maintaining gains made during the preparatory period. In this case, the intensity would be 80-

85% of 1 RM with a corresponding volume of 2-3 sets of 6-8 repetitions. Ultimately, intensity and volume is shaped by input from the coaching staff, the current game schedule, the physical status of the athlete(s), and the ongoing evaluation of performance goals. It is important to avoid overtraining during this phase, as it will negatively affect performance. During this period, the primary emphasis is placed on skill training and practice for the desired competition.

The aforementioned phases also correspond to the different athletic seasons. The preparatory phase encompasses the majority of the off-season and the entire pre-season. Meanwhile, the competitive phase runs throughout the in-season for each particular sport. For example, the competitive phase for high school football lasts during the entire ten game regular season, as well as any playoff games. Throughout the in-season, it is necessary to consistently adjust the microcycles based on injury, rehabilitation, fatigue, mental sharpness, and performance.

Now that you have a basic understanding of periodization, I must discuss the differences between linear and nonlinear (undulating) periodization. Classic or linear periodization involves consistent, deliberate manipulation of volume and intensity based on the phases discussed earlier. The volume (reps and sets) is consistent from one day to the next in this approach. In contrast, undulating models usually have different volumes and intensities from one day to the next. For example, an athlete may do 3 sets of 8-12 reps on Monday, while performing 5 sets of 3-5 reps on the next training day (Wednesday). Which method is better? Research supports both. One benefit of undulating periodization may be the absence of neural fatigue brought about by perpetual, increasing intensities linked to the linear model.[21] On the other hand, supporters of the linear model contest that the high relative levels of daily intensity involved with non-linear training may quickly result in overtraining.[19] I suggest that whatever model you choose you carefully consider short-term, intermediate and long-term goals, in addition to your own physical capabilities and limitations.

After digesting all of this information regarding periodization, you may be wondering how this affects the average person interested in getting in better shape. Whether you are a weekend warrior or simply going to the gym three times per week, you can apply these principles to your training regimen. Remember, the body adapts quickly to stress we place on it. Therefore, it is important to constantly evaluate and modify your training to avoid mental boredom, physical plateaus, and eventually disappointment and frustration with your lack of progress toward your goals. Many people set out to lose weight and get fit every year. However, they often fail due to poor planning, lack of accountability, inconsistency and, perhaps most importantly, improper progression. Most people get stuck doing the same exercises on the same days with the same number of sets and reps. Eventually, they lose interest and motivation, which in turn may lead to quitting the exercise program altogether. Yet, I believe a carefully constructed plan, established to meet specific goals at specific times, will transform your body. This strategy of changing volume and intensity will work for the individual trying to lose fifty pounds in one year or the forty-year-old recreational skier planning for a winter trip to Colorado.

In conclusion, I encourage you to consider implementing the concepts of periodization in your fitness routine. Although it may seem complicated, I assure you that simply applying some of the basic principles to your exercise regimen will bring a positive change to your workouts and prevent accommodation and training plateaus. More importantly, structuring your training in this manner will ensure proper progression at intensity levels that create positive physical adaptations and maximize performance. Through this scientific approach, you can prevent injury and develop a blueprint for success. This plan offers a sound framework allowing you flexibility within your training, but it also directs your training choices and provides a logical progression to ensure peak performance at critical times during the year. Failing to plan is planning to fail. So, if you are interested in maximizing your training, it is essential to follow a periodized training program.

Brian Schiff, P.T., CSCS

The Fitness Edge
5130 Bradenton Avenue, Suite B
Dublin, Ohio 43017
614-761-9242
Brian.Schiff@thepowerofchampions.com
www.thefitnessedge.cc

SECTION FIVE
The Heart of A Champion

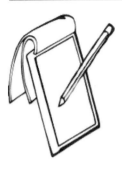

Notes from Phil

Mark Twain said, "One learns people through the heart, not the eyes or the intellect." Beyond the type of "heart" that relates to attitude, which we've already addressed, and beyond the intangible "heart" referred to by Twain, we need to recognize the virtue of the other type of "heart." That noble, ever-working muscle does its best to deliver oxygen to every cell in your body, and while we live in a nation where many focus on the mirror, we, as Champions, have to concern ourselves with that vital internal pump.

We begin this section with Champion Brett Pruitt instructing you on the finer points of exercise intensity, teaching you to use your "heart" as a gauge. Renowned researcher, Champion Wayne Westcott, then takes the baton to reveal what research has uncovered about strength training and the cardiovascular system.

Ya gotta have heart! Champions always do!

Putting Your Heart into Your Exercise Program by Brett A. Pruitt

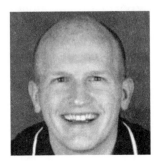

Champion Brett A. Pruitt of Longmont, Colorado, Exercise Physiologist and Master Trainer, holds numerous certifications and presents worldwide. Brett's education, experience, knowledge and fun approach to health and wellness make him a highly sought-after fitness professional.

Most exercisers have heard of the term "training heart rate" or "target heart zone" (THZ), and many of you have seen the heart rate charts up on the wall of your fitness club or aerobics studio.

However, when asked to explain what this 'mysterious' training rate really means, many individuals respond with something like, "I..., um..., well, it's the level you are supposed to be at when you workout." While this is somewhat true, there is a lot more science to it than just being an arbitrary or magical number. In order to optimize the results of your fitness program, it is very simple to calculate your own personal THZ and to understand the basics of why it is important to exercise within your proper heart rate range.

Simply put, your exercising heart rate is a percentage range within which your heart should work during a cardiovascular, or aerobic, exercise session. Cardiovascular exercise helps to decrease your risk of coronary heart disease, burns calories, strengthens your heart musculature and your respiratory system. Based upon recommendations from the American College of Sports Medicine (ACSM), the leading source for guidelines and research on safe and effective exercise programs, you should perform 20 to 60 minutes of continuous or intermittent aerobic exercise 3 to 5 days per week within your training heart rate zone. Your heart rate during these exercise sessions should be 60 to 85 percent of your maximal heart rate, depending upon your current fitness level and your desired results.

It is recommended that individuals who are deconditioned keep their heart rate near the minimum recommended exercising heart rate of 55-60%, or even lower, until they can maintain the recommended exercise frequency of 3 times per week for 15 to 20 minutes each time. Once you can maintain a baseline level, you can increase the intensity of the exercise. On the other hand, if your heart rate is over the recommended higher limit of 85%, it is recommended you decrease the exercise level and/or resistance gradually until your heart rate returns to an appropriate cardiovascular rate. Regardless of the intensity percentage you are working at, it is best not to stop quickly, unless you feel that you must. Try to keep moving even if it is just at a slow pace. Remember to do an appropriate cool down.

Once a basic level of cardiovascular fitness has been achieved, you should try not to let your heart rate drop below the minimum exercise rate of 60%, or you will not benefit from the exercise and the time you are putting into your workouts. During cool down, you should continue to exercise, but at a lower intensity until your heart rate drops to approximately 120 beats per minute, so as not to cause a blood pooling effect that could lead to dizziness and/or fainting. The cool down can also help loosen any muscular cramps you may have.

So how do you determine your specific training heart rate range? For each individual there is an intensity of exercise which is enough to condition the cardiovascular system and the muscles, is not overly strenuous and leads to physical fitness.

Calculating Your Exercise Target Heart Rate Zone

There is a relationship between your age, resting heart rate, and maximal aerobic power. Assuming you are healthy, you can use the following formula, referred to as the Heart Rate Reserve (HRR), or Karvonen, method. It can be used to determine your THZ based upon the ACSM guidelines:

A.   Age: _____
B.   Age predicted Maximum Heart Rate:
       220-Age=   _____
C.   Resting Heart Rate*   _____
D.   B - C =   _____
E.   D x 0.60 =   _____
F.   D x 0.85 =   _____
G.   C + E =   _____

This is your approximate MINIMUM Exercise Heart Rate.

H.   C + F =   _____

This is your approximate MAXIMUM Exercise Heart Rate.

*Resting Heart Rate should be taken for a full minute first thing in the morning prior to getting out of bed. Take it for three consecutive days and average the results.

Below 60%, you will achieve little increase in aerobic capacity. However, remember depending upon your current fitness level, if you are deconditioned, exercising below 60% may be appropriate. Exercising above 85% provides little added cardiovascular benefit, as most individuals begin transitioning into anaerobic energy production at this intensity, which is not essential unless you are training for specific sports-performance related results.

To determine whether you are in your target heart zone, you will have to learn how to count your exercise heart rate, or pulse, if you do not have a heart rate monitor. It is important to count your pulse both during the workout, to see if you are in your training zone, and at the end of the workout, to make sure you have cooled down properly. You can find your pulse on the side of your neck or at the wrist at the base of your thumb. Use light pressure with the first two fingers of the opposite hand. Do not use the thumb as you can actually get a double, or false, reading. Practice finding your heart rate at rest and count the beats in a ten-second period. Multiply this number by six to obtain your beats per minute (bpm). Now you are ready to monitor your heart rate during exercise.

You should measure your heart rate about five to ten minutes into your exercise routine and about every 10 to 15 minutes thereafter. Upon slowing down or stopping exercise, your heart rate should normally lower fairly quickly. Within three minutes after exercise, your pulse should be below 120 bpm; five minutes after, it should be below 100 bpm. If your heart rate does not lower to these levels in the relative timeframes, the exercise level may have been too difficult or you may have specific health considerations to discuss with your physician.

As you become comfortable with taking your pulse and determining your THZ, you can also use a technique called "perceived exertion." That is, once you know how it "feels" when you are working in your target heart zone, you can estimate your exertion level without taking your pulse as frequently. You should feel like you are working slightly harder than is comfortable, and yet you should be able to speak easily in short sentences without gasping for air. This is often referred to as the "talk test."

Use the Exercise Target Heart Rate Zone formula as part of your gauge to determine the heart rate range you should aim for during an aerobic workout. Once again, it is recommended that you work somewhere in your lower range during the first month of your training. Your personal trainer or fitness instructor can help you with specific training goals and applications. As with any exercise program, you should always contact your physician first to make sure that there are no special exceptions, considerations, or reasons that you should not take part in a given exercise program or routine.

Remember, fitness can be fun when you put your heart into it!

Brett A. Pruitt, M.S., PFT

1-2-1 Personal Training
428 Sumner St.
Longmont CO 80501
303-485-8092
Brett.Pruitt@thepowerofchampions.com

Strength Training and Blood Pressure: The Heart of the Matter by Wayne L. Westcott

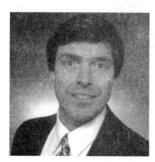

Champion Wayne L. Westcott of Quincy, Massachusetts is the fitness research director at South Shore YMCA in Quincy, Massachusetts, and author of 19 fitness books as well as certification textbook chapters for NSCA, ACE and YMCA of the USA.

Over the past several years, numerous research studies have clearly demonstrated that sensible strength training is an essential physical activity for middle-aged and older adults.

Regular resistance exercise has been shown to provide important health and fitness benefits for both the musculoskeletal system and the cardiovascular system, as well as to reduce the risk of various degenerative and debilitating diseases.[22]

Unfortunately, many of the men and women who have the most to gain from a strength training program are least likely to do so. Leading their litany of reasons for avoiding this physical activity is the unfounded fear that resistance exercise produces adverse affects on blood pressure. Somehow, they have heard that strength training spikes blood pressure to dangerous levels during exercise execution and that it raises resting blood pressure beyond safe limits over time.

While improperly performed resistance exercise can indeed be problematic in this regard, be assured that sensible strength training is not harmful to blood pressure during or after the workout. In fact, research reveals that well-designed strength training programs are just as beneficial for blood pressure as aerobic exercise programs.[23, 24] On the contrary, there is much research that indicates beneficial blood pressure adaptations to sensible strength exercise.[25, 26]

Keep in mind that people with certain medical conditions (e.g., uncontrolled hypertension, aneurism) should not perform resistance exercise; that certain resistance training actions (e.g., breath holding, isometric holding) can raise blood pressure readings beyond recommended levels; and that exercise participants should always follow their physician's guidelines regarding strength training. With this precaution, consider some of the studies we have conducted on blood pressure response to resistance exercise. These will be addressed in three separate categories:

Immediate Blood Pressure Response - This represents the blood pressure change during performance of a strength exercise.

Short-Term Blood Pressure Response - This represents the blood pressure change at the end of a strength training session.

Long-Term Blood Pressure Response - This represents the blood pressure change at the completion of a strength training program (8 to 10 weeks).

Immediate Blood Pressure Response to Strength Exercise

In 1983, the YMCA and the New England Cardiovascular Health Institute teamed up to assess blood pressure changes in 24 men and women (mean age 38 years) as they performed 10 dumbbell curls with the heaviest weight load possible.[27] The study revealed a 34 percent increase in systolic blood pressure, which represents a normal cardiovascular response to vigorous physical activity and is well below the 225 mm Hg caution level for exercise systolic readings recommended by the American College of Sports Medicine.[28]

Because lower body strength training involves more muscle mass and force production than upper body strength training, we later conducted a similar study with 25 men and women (mean age 38 years) as they performed 10 leg presses with the heaviest weight load possible.[29] In this instance, there was a 50 percent increase in systolic blood pressure, which represents a normal cardiovascular response to vigorous physical activity and is below the 225 mm Hg caution level for exercise systolic readings established by the American College of Sports Medicine.[28]

Generally speaking, the systolic blood pressure response to properly performed strength training (continuous breathing, continuous movement, appropriate weight loads) is similar to the systolic blood pressure response during endurance exercise. Research with 23 men and women revealed a 35 percent increase in systolic blood pressure during a 20-minute session of stationary cycling at 75 percent of maximum heart rate.[30]

When you perform strength exercise or aerobic activity, your heart beats faster (increased heart rate) and harder (increased systolic blood pressure) to pump more oxygen-rich blood to the working muscles. Your circulatory system adjusts accordingly by dilating blood vessels and opening additional capillaries to accommodate greater and more forceful blood flow, which is why the research subjects' diastolic blood pressure readings remained the same or decreased during performance of the exercise set.

Short-Term Blood Pressure Response to Strength Exercise

Because typical strength training sessions involve several resistance exercises, we investigated the short-term effects on blood pressure following a circuit of 11 weight stack machines.[31] The 100 men and women (mean age 37 years) in this study performed each exercise for one set of 8 to 12 repetitions to temporary muscle fatigue. Basically, the subjects' post-exercise blood pressure readings were the same as their pre-exercise blood pressure readings, indicating excellent cardiovascular system adaptations to a standard circuit strength training session.

Recently, we examined the short-term blood pressure response to a strength training session more closely.[32] In this study, 140 men and women (mean age 57 years) were assessed for blood pressure at rest and approximately one minute after completing a circuit of 12 weight stack machines (one set of 8 to 12 repetitions to temporary muscle fatigue). These beginning exercisers were assessed during the third, sixth and ninth week of an introductory strength training program. The subjects experienced progressively greater reductions in their pre- to post-workout systolic blood pressure readings every three weeks throughout the training period (1.2 mm Hg, 2.5 mm Hg and 4.5 mm Hg). These findings suggest positive and progressive cardiovascular system adaptations to successive strength training sessions with respect to systolic blood pressure response.

Diastolic blood pressure readings did not show a similar pattern of pre-to-post workout decrease. However, the subjects recorded a 6.3 mm Hg mean reduction in systolic blood pressure and a 2.2 mm Hg mean reduction in diastolic blood pressure over the course of the 10-week training period.

Long-Term Blood Pressure Response to Strength Exercise

Blood pressure changes that occur over a period of weeks, such as those noted above, represent what we consider long-term responses to the strength training program. One of the larger studies on the long-term blood pressure response to strength training was conducted at the South Shore YMCA.[33] A total of 785 men and women participated in this study, which included 25 minutes of strength exercise and 25 minutes of aerobic activity, two or three days a week for a period of eight weeks. Mean resting blood pressure for subjects between 21 and 40 years old decreased 4.5 mm Hg systolic and 3.2 mm Hg diastolic; mean resting blood pressure for subjects between 41 and 60 years old decreased 2.5 mm Hg systolic and 2.4 mm Hg diastolic; and mean resting blood pressure for subjects between 61 and 80 years old decreased 6.2 mm Hg systolic and 3.7 mm Hg diastolic. These statistically significant results suggest that a basic program of strength and endurance exercise may be highly effective for reducing resting blood pressure in adults of all ages.

A later study with 77 senior golfers (mean age 57 years) revealed similar blood pressure responses following eight weeks of strength exercise only.[34] These subjects performed one set of 8 to 12 repetitions on 13 weight stack machines, three days per week for the two month training period. Their mean systolic blood pressure decreased 7.4 mm Hg, and their mean diastolic blood pressure decreased 2.7 mm Hg.

Summary

Based on the studies reviewed, it would seem that sensible strength training does not have detrimental effects on blood pressure in medically cleared men and women between 20 and 80 years of age. In fact, both the short-term and long-term responses to properly performed strength exercise appear to be beneficial, with temporarily lower blood pressure readings after the exercise session and permanently lower blood pressure readings after eight to 10 weeks of regular training. In addition, the systolic blood pressure elevation experienced during a 10 repetition-maximum set of strength exercise is similar to that experienced during standard aerobic activity, and is well within the normal response range established by the American College of Sports Medicine.

Recommendations for Sensible Strength Training

Most of the research showing beneficial blood pressure adaptations to regular resistance exercise involved circuit strength training programs. This time efficient type of strength training requires relatively more activity time and less recovery time than standard multiple-set exercise protocols. Generally performed on a line of 10 to 15 resistance machines, circuit strength training involves a set of exercise for a specific muscle group, followed by a set of exercise for a different muscle group, and so on, until all of the major muscle groups have been effectively addressed within a 20 to 30 minute time period.

A sample circuit strength training workout might feature one set of 8 to 12 repetitions on the following dozen resistance machines: (1) leg extension; (2) leg curl; (3) hip adduction; (4) hip abduction; (5) leg press; (6) chest cross; (7) back pullover; (8) lateral raise; (9) triceps extension; (10) biceps curl; (11) lower back extension; and (12) abdominal curl. Each exercise set should be performed with proper posture, correct breathing and controlled repetitions.

Suggestions for sensible strength training include the following performance guidelines:

- Use weight loads that can be performed with correct exercise technique for at least eight controlled repetitions.
- Breathe continuously throughout each exercise set, exhaling during the lifting actions and inhaling during the lowering actions.
- Move the weight load continuously throughout each exercise set, taking about two seconds for the lifting actions and about four seconds for the lowering actions.
- Use relatively loose handgrips whenever possible.
- Keep the face and neck muscles as relaxed as possible throughout each exercise set.
- Train regularly with sufficient recovery time (48 to 96 hours) between successive exercise sessions.

Wayne L. Westcott, Ph.D., CSCS

Fitness Research Director
South Shore YMCA
79 Coddington Street
Quincy, MA 02169
617-479-8500
Wayne.Westcott@thepowerofchampions.com

SECTION SIX
Eat Like a Champion

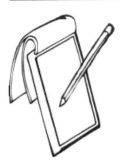

Notes from Phil

In this section, the Champions have their greatest challenge. They're going to talk to you about food. Why is this so challenging? Allow me to send you to the supermarket . . . .not necessarily to shop, but to stand by the checkout counter and study the magazine rack. Every magazine has "diet tips," "nutritional secrets," "fat loss recipes," or "the tricks that helped Midwest Mary lose 60 pounds for her wedding." Start to pick up the magazines and flip through the articles. I defy you to come up with even a single point that is present in every one of the articles.

One will sing the praises of a low-carb lifestyle. Another will tell you to avoid fat. Another will teach you to cut calories, while another promises calories are good, if consumed in the right food combinations.

This is the area where people are most confused, and as certified Personal Fitness Trainers, it is not our primary or our documented area of expertise. Still, without the supportive nutrition component in place, all physical improvement efforts will fall short. Our challenge, therefore, is to provide real-world nutritional information that provides not a specific diet regimen, but rather clarity. What you'll find as you read through this section is that there are some foundational elements of supportive eating that Champions share and, unlike the magazine articles, there isn't any conflict. Our Champions have personally helped tens of thousands of people find the fitness or weight loss results they sought after, and when all nutritional notes are compared, the similarity in the approach leads to clear evidence that "the Champions know what works."

In this section, Champion Jason Robertson opens by explaining why you shouldn't put detrimental foods into your body any more than you'd want to fill your automobile gas tank with water. Champion Billy Beck III will then help you understand why eating frequently becomes a vital part of the process, whether you seek muscle gain, energy increase, or a systemic metabolic boost leading to ongoing fat reduction. Champion Kelly Huggins will provide further clarity as he helps you understand why, despite a societal pull to "eat less to weigh less," significant amounts of the right types of foods keep metabolism revved in high gear.

Champion Maryellen Jordan provides clarity as to how sugar impacts your body and how modifying sugar intake can have a massive payoff. Champion Brian Calkins continues on the sugar theme by helping you understand the difference between complex carbs and simple sugars, and then Champion Paul Ohashi provides some real world ideas for "curing the sugar-holic."

Next on the agenda, Champion Kevin Gendron plays up the value of the most vital, yet probably the most neglected nutrient, and the section continues with Brad Schoenfeld helping to shed some light on the trend that leads millions to "just cut carbs."

Champion John Spencer Ellis provides the finishing touch by sharing valuable insight into what has evolved into the most popular supplement among athletes, creatine.

Be prepared to let go of some long-held false beliefs, and enter into a realm where "diet" no longer means "deprivation." A supportive "diet" means fueling the body efficiently and with premium fuel. You'll be amazed how dramatically your body can change. Let's get started . . .

The Right Nutrition by Jason Robertson

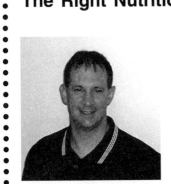

Champion Jason ('JJ') Robertson of Pittsburgh, Pennsylvania is the owner of Exercise Expressions, a premier Fitness Studio in western Pennsylvania offering Personal Training and fitness classes. With over 10 years of experience, JJ brings a diverse approach to fitness from education, athletics and the Marine Corps.

Let's start this chapter with a question. Are you happy with the way you look and feel?

Anything you put into your body will in part determine how you look and feel. Do you consume sugar, white flour, fatty foods or alcohol on a regular basis? What you consume will determine what you see in the mirror. If your car were running low on fuel, would you fill up the gas tank with water? No! Because it would have a detrimental effect on your vehicle. Is your body any less important? Just as you would not put water into the gas tank of your vehicle, do not put inefficient fuel into your own body. You should attempt to eat right.

Just Eat Right!

We all know we should eat right. So why don't we? After you make a commitment to eating right, what do you do? How do you define "The Right Nutrition?" You could go to your local bookstore. But which top-selling book would you buy? One book says, "Fat is evil! Stay away from fat! Carbohydrates give you fuel and energy." Another book claims, "Carbohydrates are evil! Stay away from carbs! You need fat to burn fat!" Before you realize what has happened, you'll be in the "self-help" section seeking inner peace. It is a very confusing world out there in the "Eat Right Land."

In order to facilitate a positive change, you need to begin with a new paradigm of thinking. At some level food is fuel. We are biological beings with biological needs. Just as your vehicle requires gasoline to run effectively, food provides fuel for your body.

What kind of fuel do you require? The human body, this means you, requires 6 basic nutrients. These nutrients include proteins, carbohydrates, fats, vitamins, minerals and water. This is the reason we eat food, to supply the body with these 6 basic nutrients.

Supportive Eating

If you are currently following a diet that limits calories or neglects basic nutrients, it will fail. Providing your body with the basic nutrients in the right nutrition program will allow for optimal recovery, energy, growth and support your metabolism. One of the easiest ways to "overtrain" is simply by "under recovery" or not eating supportively. You could workout for hours each day, as if your life depended on it, but if your nutrition program doesn't provide your body with the proper nutrients, you could be wasting your time and energy, or worse, losing muscle and gaining fat!

How do you supply your body with these 6 basic nutrients? By eating what we call "supportively." Supportive eating describes an effective nutrition program that provides all 6 basic nutrients. How do you do that?

Protein and Carbs

Every 3 to 3 1/2 hours eat a small, well-balanced meal containing a lean protein, a starchy carbohydrate and a fibrous carbohydrate. Each meal should be low in fat, low in sugar and free from processed or refined foods. Choose foods that are as natural and wholesome as possible. This means 6 – 7 supportive meals a day as opposed to what most of us are accustomed to. But let me ask you this, did the last "diet" you followed give you the lasting results you had hoped for? Probably not! The definition of insanity is doing the same thing over and over again and expecting different results. Champion Billy Beck III shares his client's success in this regard in his chapter, 'The Benefits of Frequent Eating.' This formula gets results!

When you look at your dinner plate, you should be able to divide the plate into equal thirds. The three divisions on the plate allow you to visualize equal compartments for a lean protein, a starchy carbohydrate and a fibrous carbohydrate. A lean protein may be any white fish, egg whites, chicken breast, tuna, shrimp, lobster, soybeans, turkey breast or any meat product, which is "lean."

Recognize and avoid simple sugars, white flour, or other processed and refined carbs

Try to limit any carbohydrate containing white sugar, simple sugars or white flour. The carbohydrates you want to consume are complex carbohydrates, both fibrous and starchy. A fibrous carbohydrate is basically any vegetable item such as salad greens, broccoli, spinach, kale, carrots, cauliflower, etc. Fruits are fibrous carbs also, however, we tend to limit them, not because of the nutrients they contain, but because of the fructose or fruit sugar they contain. Fruits and fruit juices are healthy, but if you are attempting to get lean, limit their consumption. Starchy carbohydrates include brown rice, yams, potatoes, oatmeal, whole grains and other grain items that have not been processed through milling.

Champion Brian Calkins explains how to identify the different types of carbs in his chapter, 'Simple Sugars vs. Complex Carbs.'

Recognize and limit fats

Fats are a combination of carbon, hydrogen, and oxygen molecules, which form chains. Different combinations of these chains form different types of fat, including:

- saturated
- unsaturated
- hydrogenated
- essential fatty acids (EFAs)

A fat that holds as many hydrogens as it can is '**saturated**,' having no open areas where additional hydrogen molecules can bond. **Unsaturated fats**, on the other hand, have places where hydrogens are missing. There are two classses of unsaturated fats - monounsaturated and polyunsaturated.

Saturation will affect the temperature at which a fat will melt. Saturated fats are solid at room temperature, i.e., butter. Typically, if a fat is more liquid than solid at room temperature, it is an unsaturated fat.

You want to limit or avoid saturated fats. The following unsaturated fats are healthier choices:

- canola oil
- corn oil
- olive oil
- peanut oil
- safflower oil
- soybean oil
- vegetable oil

Hydrogenated fats are 'man-made.' Food processors force hydrogen into an unsaturated fat to saturate it in order to change its consistency and help keep the food fresher, longer. As a result, the fat is no longer a healthy food choice. Hydrogenated fats are found in snack foods, chips, and other processed foods.

Essential Fatty Acids - Whenever you see the word 'essential' in a nutritional context, it means that the substance is something that the body is incapable of making and must be obtained from the foods we eat. Essential Fatty Acids (EFAs) are the raw materials your body needs to build cells and keep skin, hair, and joints healthy. They can be found in fish products and oils such as primrose, flaxseed, canola and safflower. Following a supportive nutrition program and eating a variety of lean protein, starchy and fibrous carbs should fulfill your EFA requirements.

Your best bet is to become an educated consumer and learn how to read and understand food labels so that you can make the healthiest, most nutritious choices possible. If you are unsure about a fat, put some in a clear container in the refrigerator. The clearer it remains, the more unsaturated it is. If it is hard at room temperature, it's a saturated fat.

Drink Water Daily

One of the 6 basic nutrients we have not yet addressed is water. I urge you to drink clean, fresh water throughout the day. I learned the benefits of water consumption in the Marine Corps. The Marines who did not drink water continuously struggled in the fitness and recovery component of their training. When forced to consume water, the immediate results were astounding. Other drinks count toward your water; however, you should limit drinks with caffeine and simple sugars. Read Champion Kevin Gendron's chapter, 'Hydration,' for practical advice in this regard.

Meals and Snack Meals

New clients often ask, "I understand what I should be eating for my meals, but what would be a good snack?" Get the concept of "snack vs. meal" out of your vocabulary. If your car is running on fumes, do you pull into the gas station and put in $2 worth of gas? Why then would you only put in a measly amount of fuel into your own body when you are running low on fuel? Think of each meal as an opportunity to fuel your body with proper nutrients. Ideally, each meal should be equally balanced. This means you are consuming 6-7 equal meals each day. Think in terms of Meal 1, Meal 2, and so on. When someone asks you, "What did you eat for lunch?," your answer should be along these lines, "Well, Meal 4 was a whole wheat pita stuffed with tuna, lettuce and tomato. I guess that was my lunch."

How Much Should You Eat?

The simplicity of the right nutrition program is you are not relying on counting portions or calories. When you eat supportively, calories are used to support metabolism and feed muscles, which in turn leaves few calories to be stored as body fat. With your entire nutrient needs being met, your body will tell you how much to consume. You should never be "stuffed" after a meal or feel "starving" before a meal. If you are still hungry between meals, you should increase the portion sizes of each meal component. If you are one of those people who just has to know how much to eat, find a 6" plate. Divide the plate into thirds; fill one third with a lean protein, one with a starchy carbohydrate and the last with a fibrous carbohydrate. As your metabolism increases, get an 8" plate and apply the same technology.

How do you eat right when you have a job, are raising kids or are a "busy person?" First realize this is just a single step in a new direction. You don't need to be perfect, just better. Find ways to prepare food ahead of time. You can always have vegetables such as carrots, celery or salad greens ready to go. If you can't eat a supportive meal, instead of skipping a meal, turn to a good quality supplement bar or protein shake. Remember: Food First, Supplements Second!

Be patient with yourself. Seek progression and not perfection. Just do a little bit better today than you did yesterday and you will constantly improve.

Jason Robertson, CPT NSCA, AIFE, IFPA, CSN IFPA, Parrillo Performance Master Trainer
CCAC Weight Training Instructor

Exercise Expressions
3220 Washington Road
McMurray, PA 15317
724-492-4776
Jason.Robertson@thepowerofchampions.com
www.ExerciseExpressions.com

The Benefits of Frequent Eating by Billy Beck III

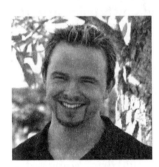

Champion Billy Beck III of Fort Lauderdale, Florida is the Fitness Director of GetCYCED! Fitness where he leads the Best Training Team in the Nation and has helped thousands change their bodies and lives in dramatic fashion.

Just the other day, I was watching ESPN 2 and I was amazed at what I saw before me. SUMO WRESTLING!

"Whoa, those guys must eat all day!!!" was my first thought. "Heck, the winner must eat the loser. I can't believe how much fat these guys put on." Then I got a great idea. I realized that sumo wrestlers were great at exactly the opposite of what most people want. Being big and fat! So I figured that it was important to know what sumos do and to avoid it at all costs. So I dug in and did some research and I could not believe what I found.

You would think that these massive men eat all day, at least 6 meals. However, that is not the case. The typical day for a sumo consists of getting up at the crack of dawn, around 6 a.m., and immediately working out for four hours and eating only two meals per day![35] On average, a sumo today tips the scales at 339 pounds.[36] With four hours of exercise and only two meals per day, it is hard to conceive how these men get so obese.

Now compare this to the typical American's lifestyle. In today's fast-paced world most of us struggle to find the time to exercise and eat often. Most people often skip breakfast, maybe grab a sandwich or a salad for lunch and get home at night ravenous. At this point, it is unlikely that anyone will eat a "sensible" meal. The American lifestyle is quite similar to that of a sumo wrestler and, unfortunately, it shows. America is the fattest nation on the planet with almost 70% of our population classified as overweight. The most obvious similarity is the infrequency of meals. Traditionally, we think that to lose fat we must eat less. Let's take a closer look at how the human body reacts.

First of all, it is important to understand that your body can only deal with a certain amount of food at a time. When too much food is ingested, unused food is stored as fat or, if you possess a fast metabolism, the excess will be burned off as heat. The average sumo wrestler ingests approximately 5,000 calories in only two meals while the much leaner average Japanese consumes about 2,279 calories per day divided into three meals.[37] Thus, we can conclude that one of the factors of the sumos' large size, and the majority of Americans, is their consumption of large, infrequent meals.[38]

When your body is fed small meals throughout the day, it reacts quite differently. In fact, when eating small, supportive meals every 3-3 ½ hours, your metabolism naturally speeds up and puts your body in a state where it can release fat for fuel 24 hours a day, 7 days per week. The majority of people who I meet are often eating only 1 to 3 meals per day and, despite their best efforts in the gym, they are not seeing results.

Allow me to introduce you to Denise. When I met Denise, she was doing aerobics classes five days per week for an hour and half at a time. At the age of forty eight, Denise's weight had slowly crept up to 160 pounds - the heaviest she had ever been in her life.

A typical day for Denise started at 7 a.m. with a cup of coffee. She was out the door at 8 a.m. to catch her daily step class. She would go home and shower and maybe run some errands in the morning and often skipped lunch or, if she had time, she would get a small turkey sub with a diet coke. Her afternoons were spent at the office following up on orders and other projects.

Denise loves to cook and she prepared dinner for her husband every night. She would drink some red wine as she cooked dinner, which was nothing short of a small feast. It usually consisted of a main entrée of chicken, fish or beef with potatoes, rice or pasta and a big salad with dressing. Dinner sounds all right except for the serving sizes. Since she had not eaten all day, she was starving and ate until she was not just satisfied but stuffed to the gills!

In looking at Denise's lifestyle at the time, our first step was to bring in the missing components of the "Synergy." We added resistance training to her morning workout while reducing the duration of her aerobic exercise. Denise was hesitant about cutting back on her aerobic exercise and when I told her about eating more often, she, well, freaked out. "I can't do that! I will blow up like a whale!!! Are you crazy?!!!" I quickly responded, "Just trust me." (By the look on her face I could tell that the "Just-trust-me line" was not going to cut it.) I told her, "Denise, I know how you feel because the majority of my clients in your situation felt the exact same way when I told them to eat more often. But what they found was that by eating supportive meals consisting of visibly equal portions of lean protein, starchy carbohydrates and fibrous vegetables every 3-3 ½ hours every one of them noticed a positive change in the way they looked and felt.

"There is a series of signs that will let you know that it's working. The first sign you will notice is that you have more energy. Next, you will be eating more food than ever without gaining weight. This is an indication that your body's ability to burn through food is greatly enhanced (aka faster metabolism). Then you will notice that your clothes will begin to fit looser. And finally, you will see things visibly tighten up. So, Denise, does that sound like something you would like to try?"

She agreed and over the course of a few weeks she went from her usual 1-2 meals per day to 5-6 meals daily. After only four months of eating more often and bringing the Synergy together, Denise went from 160 pounds all the way down to a lean and toned 117. At the age of forty eight, Denise was in the best shape of her life and even took her "after" photo in her sixteen-year-old niece's bikini!

If you keep doing the same things, you will keep getting the same things. In order for things to change, you must change. Eating balanced meals frequently throughout the day is a pivotal step in speeding metabolism and allowing you to live in the body that you desire and deserve.

Billy Beck III, NSCA, ACE, NASM, Fitness Institute International

954-915-0080
Billy.Beck@thepowerofchampions.com

Burn Fat by Eating More! by Kelly Huggins

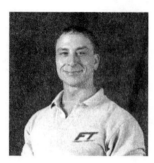

Champion Kelly Huggins of Marietta, Georgia owns a Fitness Together personal training studio that serves the metro Atlanta area. Degreed in Exercise Science, Kelly can help you when it is difficult losing weight or keeping it off.

I remember when I was in high school chemistry class the teacher had us take a potato chip and burn it.

Though it took a few seconds, the chip burst into flames and disintegrated. The purpose of this exercise was to demonstrate the First Law of Thermodynamics.

The First Law of Thermodynamics states that energy can neither be created nor destroyed – only converted from one form to another. When we eat food, we are basically transforming food into energy for our body. In order to do that, we use energy to break down the food. Kind of ironic, isn't it? We measure this energy in kilocalories, or to make it simple, just calories.

Now, here is the kicker. Not all calories are the same. We can't argue that 1 calorie doesn't equal 1 calorie. It does. That's like asking, "What weighs more, a ton of feathers or a ton of bricks?" However, the amount of energy that is needed to break down different food substances that have the same amount of calories can vary greatly.

To give you an example, I want you to think of the difference between burning a piece of cardboard and a piece of wood. Imagine that they are equal in the amount of "calories" they have. Which would burn faster, the cardboard or the piece of wood? Even though they both have the same amount of energy, the cardboard will burn much faster. Why? Because the amount of energy released in heat does not have to be as great. It simply breaks down easier.

Just like that potato chip I mentioned earlier, it burned up quickly. Try taking a piece of raw broccoli and doing the same thing; you will have to stand there and hold the flame to it. (But don't try this, please take my word for it.) Compare the potato chip to the broccoli - which do you think will digest faster?

The Mistakes We Have Made

Unfortunately, we have been fooled into believing that depriving ourselves of food (that is calories) will optimize our weight loss efforts. We hear this from weight-loss centers, infomercials, and magazines. Weight loss might be initially achieved, but weight is nothing more than gravity pulling an object toward Earth. Most of the initial weight you lose is water and stored food in the digestive tract. Once you start decreasing the carbohydrate energy, you begin utilizing proteins as fuel. By eating less, it's really not fat you're losing but muscle and everything else that is important.

Now, what does this really mean? It means you need to eat regularly throughout the day to keep burning calories efficiently. As Phil says, it's Supportive Eating. You see, by eating regular meals throughout the day you are constantly providing fuel to your metabolism, your body. This keeps the thermogenic engines burning. However, you still have to eat the right kinds of food with the right consistency. Even if your caloric intake is low, when you eat hamburgers, French fries, and Pop-Tarts as the staple of your diet, you are going to have problems.

Understanding the Thermic Effect of Food

Before I go any further and explain what you need to do, I want to define thermogenesis, or the thermic effect of food. The thermic effect of food is the amount of energy (calories) needed to digest, absorb, transport and store food. The amount of calories you use on average can range between 10-25% of the calories ingested. How often you eat and what kind of food you eat has an impact on how many calories are used. For example, when you eat lean protein, you can utilize up to 35% of the calories it offers. On the other hand, when you eat a cookie the cost will be 10% or lower.

What I would like to do now is to provide you with two steps to follow when creating your dietary habits.

Step 1: How Often Should You Eat?

You probably have heard that you should eat 4-6 small meals throughout the day. This is true without exception. By eating every 3 ½-4 hours, you are supportively keeping your metabolism in check throughout the day. Do not skip breakfast. By skipping breakfast you don't kick start the metabolism. You are also more likely to eat larger, high fat meals for lunch and dinner. Small meals and snacks will prevent you from binging late in the day. You will feel satisfied, so there is no need to eat more.

By eating all day, you will maintain a much higher basal metabolic rate (the amount of calories you burn at rest). When you skip meals, especially breakfast, your body will tell itself to burn fewer calories. This is a survival mechanism the body employs when it feels that there may be a starvation period. As the metabolism slows down, the body will convert as much food into fat as possible. In this instance, the thermic effect of food is not beneficial to you. In his chapter, 'Understanding Metabolism,' Champion Dan Houston demystifies 'metabolism' to help you make healthier food choices that ultimately lead to successfully reaching your fitness goals.

Step 2: What to Eat?

First of all, there is one concept that I want you to remember: Moderation, Variety and Balance. If you get too hung up on what to eat, it can be mentally draining. You simply need to get an idea of what kinds of foods are best to eat and when it is most beneficial to eat them.

Carbohydrates, Proteins and Fats

Carbohydrates:

Carbohydrates come in 3 different forms:

- simple sugars
- complex (aka starchy) carbohydrates
- fibrous carbohydrates

Of the three, the one that has the lowest thermic effect is simple sugars. Simple sugars usually include all desserts, juice, soda, white rice, honey, and refined flour products (i.e., white bread). Avoid these as much as possible. Not only do they break down fast (which means they can easily turn to fat), but they will make you feel hungry shortly after eating them. And they have little, if any, nutrients.

Complex carbohydrates include foods like potatoes, sweet potatoes, bananas, brown rice, beans, oatmeal and whole grains. They digest more slowly and steadily than simple sugars. It is ideal to have 2-3 servings of complex carbs a day.

Fibrous carbohydrates have a very high thermic effect and utilize a lot of caloric energy. Fibrous carbohydrates include all vegetables as well most fruits and nuts, i.e., broccoli, cauliflower, apples, almonds, onions, peppers and romaine lettuce. These foods have lots of nutrients, slow down the digestive processes of other foods and aid in the digestion of protein. Champion Brian Calkins offers no nonsense guidelines to carbs in his chapter, 'Simple Sugars vs. Complex Carbs.'

Protein:

We get most of our protein from meats, dairy, eggs and, in some cases, beans and nuts. As I mentioned earlier, proteins have a high thermogenic effect. A piece of grilled chicken can utilize as much as 35% of the calories it offers. The amino acids it is composed of can also help slow down the digestive processes of carbohydrates and fat.

Fat:

Your body needs fat. Unsaturated fats are good for you in moderation. Saturated fats should be avoided altogether. In both unsaturated and saturated fats, the thermic effect will always be low. However, when combined with lean protein sources and fibrous carbohydrates, the breakdown of fat will take longer. Unfortunately, many of the foods Americans eat are very high in fat and, in some cases, are higher in fat than proteins and carbohydrates.

Here's a nutrient-rich meal plan to try:

Breakfast - Oatmeal, eggs with mushrooms and peppers
Snack - A handful of peanuts
Lunch - Grilled Chicken Salad with Romaine lettuce
Snack - Apple
Dinner - Grilled Salmon with asparagus and a small baked potato

Final Thought

As I mentioned earlier, do not get too caught up in the exact details. Just know that you need lean protein, 2-3 complex carbohydrates and lots of fibrous carbohydrates. Combine them together at meals. Eat real food. Eat the food that was grown on the ground, on a tree or was born. Don't constantly go through drive-thrus and eat stuff that comes from boxes or plastic wrappers. By making the right choices you will begin to kick your metabolism back into gear and the body fat will not only come off but stay off!

Kelly Huggins, B.S., ACSM

770-321-1347
Kelly.Huggins@thepowerofchampions.com
www.CobbFitness.com

The Impact of Sugar by Maryellen Jordan

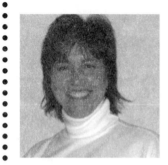

Champion Maryellen Jordan of Maumee, Ohio is the owner of Positively Fit and Fitness Specialist at a Smuckers Food Plant. For the past 12 years, she has focused on educating her clients to improve their health, fitness and well-being.

It's truly amazing how much sugar Americans consume.

Dessert after dinner, birthday cake to celebrate, chocolate to alleviate PMS symptoms, a quick 3:00 p.m. pick-me-up with a candy bar, suckers for children at the doctor's office, and ice cream cones on a hot summer day. Not to mention all the treats during the holidays. Most of these sugary foods have no significant beneficial nutrients, but supply large amounts of empty calories.

If you want something sweet to eat, it is everywhere, in schools, at work, gas stations, and in every home and restaurant in the country. In the year 2002, the average American consumed 170 pounds of sugar, 20 percent of it in the form of soda. Americans are consuming an extremely high level of refined carbohydrates that are all too readily available in our hurried lifestyles. As a result of this increased consumption of sugar and refined carbohydrates, American's waistlines have expanded in proportion.

As a child, I had a severe case of reactive hypoglycemia (low blood sugar). I received neither direction nor any nutritional advice from my medical doctor. After years of suffering with numerous, oftentimes vague and nagging symptoms I decided to take my health in my own hands. As I aged (starting about 35 years old), it became increasingly more difficult to maintain stable blood sugar levels and maintain a healthy weight with my lifelong eating habits.

So I became a student of the effect of sugar on the metabolism. Through many years of diligent research, I sought out the experts who could help me control my blood sugar successfully. I learned about the impact of sugar and the effects it had on my health. I now incorporate what I have learned and experienced about controlling blood sugar as a part of the nutrition counseling process with my clients. Mainly what I teach is back to basics - using scientifically proven ways to cut out sugar and educating clients on how to make wise food choices for the recommended 5-6 small balanced meals throughout the day.

By cutting out the sugars in your diet, you can control your insulin levels. By controlling your insulin levels, you reduce your risk of heart disease, obesity, cancer, high blood pressure, stroke and arteriosclerosis, to name just a few. You will also have more energy, feel better, look better, eliminate sweet cravings and mood swings.

So here goes. It is 3:00 p.m. You are at work, feeling sleepy, and craving something sweet. You head to the vending machine, put in your money and out comes your favorite candy bar. You eat it, within a short time your energy is up, enough to get you through your workday and home where the cycle starts all over again. So what happened? What was the impact of the sugar you just consumed? The candy bar probably had about 30 grams of sugar in it. That is equivalent to 7 ½ teaspoons of sugar. 1 teaspoon = 4 grams of sugar.

The body digested the candy bar and converted it into glucose (blood sugar), which then entered the bloodstream hopefully to be burned as energy. The problem with the candy bar is that the glucose entered the bloodstream too fast, which caused the blood sugar level to elevate.

The pancreas' response to this rapidly elevating glucose is to secrete a correspondingly high level of insulin in an attempt to transport glucose from the blood to the cells of the body. One of insulin's major roles is to decrease blood glucose levels when it gets too high. Normal levels of insulin allow the body to burn glucose for energy and store it as glycogen for future use. It is also one of your body's most effective fat storing hormones. Prolonged, elevated levels of insulin can cause the body to store glucose for future energy needs as body fat instead of generating immediate energy. The repeated consumption of high sugar foods can contribute to frequent excessive release of insulin and fat (adipose) storage.

Historically, insulin evolved as the body's mechanism to store fat in case of future famine. Primitive Ice Age ancestors could easily store fat for survival. The more fat, the more likely they would survive to childbearing age. This genetic makeup has been passed down for generations.

Our body can only store so much glucose as glycogen and what cannot be stored as glycogen will be converted to fat and stored. The buttocks, hips, back and abdomen are typical storage areas for fat. Abdominal fat has a particularly strong relationship with insulin. Elevated insulin levels can stimulate your body to store fat and prevent the body from burning fat.

Why do sugar cravings occur?

When the blood glucose level drops, and especially if it drops rapidly, cravings for foods that will raise blood glucose levels quickly are common. One of the most frequent signs of reduced blood glucose levels is a decrease in the ability to concentrate effectively. The brain needs a constant, stable supply of glucose to function. Three times each minute the brain completes a series of chemical reactions, the Krebs Cycle, in which glucose is converted into useable energy.

Ideally, insulin should be released in a series of stable, steady pulses. These pulses should occur without any dramatic spikes throughout the day. During spiking, the body can synthesize triglycerides and store body fat. The body can begin the fat synthesizing process as quickly as just two to three hours after eating sugar or any food that converts to glucose rapidly in the blood.

Just recently I had a new client come in for an initial assessment and goal setting program. She came in as a tense, anxious and very unhappy person. She had tried all different kinds of diets and they all failed her. Her goals were to lose weight, feel better and to be able to walk up stairs without her knees hurting. I sent her home with a copy of the glycemic index and her nutrition guidelines. The glycemic index ranks foods on their ability to affect blood sugar levels - the speed and degree to which food raises blood sugar. The foods have a numeric rating. The higher the index number, the faster blood sugar rises. The lower the number, the slower the food will affect the blood sugar.

The glycemic index rating depends on the type of sugar (fructose, sucrose, honey, glucose) in the food, the amount of fiber and the amount of protein and fat in the food. In addition, the manner in which the food is prepared can alter its blood sugar effect.

The next week when she came in she was a much happier person; in fact, she was elated. She had lost 6 pounds (water weight), felt happier and her knees did not hurt. She followed the nutrition guidelines and ate only from the recommended foods from the glycemic index. By doing this, she eliminated sugar and the effect of sugar from her diet in two ways. First the obvious, she eliminated the simple sugars. She also eliminated the foods from the index that turned to sugar quickly.

In general, the more processed the food, the more rapidly it can raise blood sugar levels. When you utilize the glycemic index for your food choices and eliminate most or all simple sugars and refined foods, it can contribute significantly to a more stable and balanced blood sugar.

For example, when you eat a medium-sized baked potato, especially on an empty stomach, it raises your blood sugar very rapidly. It is equivalent to having a glass of water with about 8 teaspoons of sugar. So, under the right circumstances, potatoes, even though they are a healthy food, can actually increase the rate of fat synthesis by causing a rapid elevation in blood sugar and associated elevated insulin release. To the pancreas, the source of sugar makes no difference: it will produce insulin whether the sweet is coming from the sugar bowl, a can of soda, or a piece of fruit.

Glucagon

The solution to avoiding this negative impact of sugar is to eat 5-6 small meals throughout the day balancing them with protein, low glycemic foods, and fiber. When you eat a meal that will balance your blood sugar, you can stimulate the release of the hormone glucagon which mobilizes the adipose tissue to release fat into your bloodstream so that it can be utilized as a source of energy.

Insulin and glucagon are two hormones that act in opposite ways. If you want to burn fat, you must balance these two hormones. The easiest way to maintain a stable balance between glucagon and insulin is by stabilizing your blood sugar.

Now, why did my client's knees stop hurting? We haven't even trained yet to increase the strength in her leg muscles to protect her knees. By eliminating sugar and the foods that convert to sugar rapidly from her diet, she started to stabilize the level of insulin that was being released. Excess insulin can also be a potent activator of the inflammatory process in part by signaling certain immune system cells to become more aggressive, even when that aggressiveness is not required as part of a normal healthy immune response.

What is the price we pay for consuming large quantities of sugar and high glycemic foods? We already see it in our school-aged children. Obesity, tooth decay, attention deficit disorder, hyperactivity syndromes and even Type 2 diabetes are occurring at an exponential rate. The long-term consumption of sugar and high glycemic foods is one of the surest ways to increase the risks for a number of degenerative diseases and chronic inflammatory conditions.

Unfortunately we cannot change our genetic makeup but we can control our meals and snacks to stabilize blood sugar. The use of balanced meals and snacks, the elimination of sugar, and the wise use of high glycemic foods can result in fat weight loss, more easily managed weight maintenance, improved mood, decreased food cravings, increased energy and performance and aid in the prevention of a number of health issues.

Maryellen Jordan, ACE CPT, MES

108 East Dudley Road
Maumee, Ohio 43537
419-893-5105
Maryellen.Jordan@thepowerofchampions.com

Simple Sugars vs. Complex Carbs by Brian Calkins

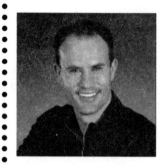

Champion Brian Calkins of Cincinnati, Ohio is recognized as a leading fitness professional in the area, Brian teaches men and women how to safely and effectively lose weight, get in shape and dramatically enhance their health, energy and vitality.

Many people seeking a positive health and fitness change are very confused about the differences between simple and complex carbohydrates.

And to make matters worse, many of the popular weight-loss solutions seem to do all they can to cloud the waters even further. My goal here is to help you understand the difference between simple sugars (aka simple carbohydrates) and complex carbohydrates, show you how they impact your health and fitness, and provide you with some simple steps you can take today to move you closer to becoming your own fitness Champion. After reading this information, you will be one critical step closer toward reaching your absolute physical best!

Carbohydrates are one of three necessary macronutrients that provide calories in our diets. The other two are protein and fat. Carbohydrates provide most of the energy needed in our daily lives, both for normal body functions (such as heartbeat, breathing, digestion, and brain activity) and for exercise (e.g., biking, walking, running up the stairs and resistance training). An ample supply of carbohydrates is absolutely necessary to sustain a healthy existence and a must if your goal is to reduce body fat and enhance your fitness level.

Carbohydrates are considered simple or complex based upon their chemical structure. Both types contain four calories per gram, and both are digested into the bloodstream as glucose, which is then used to fuel your body. The main difference between simple and complex carbs is:

Simple carbohydrates or simple sugars – These carbs are broken down and digested very quickly, but most simple carbs contain refined sugars and very few essential vitamins and minerals. Examples include table sugar, fruit juice, milk, yogurt, honey, molasses, maple syrup and brown sugar.

Complex carbohydrates – Complex carbs take longer to digest and are packed with fiber, vitamins and minerals. Examples include vegetables, whole grain breads, oatmeal, legumes, brown rice and wheat pasta.

When you eat (or drink) a simple sugar, whether it is a can of soda, a scoop of fat-free ice cream, or even a glass of orange juice, all of the ingested sugar rushes into your bloodstream resulting in a quick burst of energy. Your body promptly reacts to this sudden spike in blood sugar by calling on the pancreas to produce additional insulin to remove the excess sugar from your blood. For the moment, you have significantly lower blood sugar as a result of the insulin doing its job, resulting in a sense or feeling of needing more fuel, more energy and more calories. As you hit that residual low blood sugar, you begin to crave more of the quick-release, simple sugars, and hence you have just initiated the sugar craving cycle.

As this downward cycle continues, your pancreas continues to secrete insulin while it simultaneously reduces its production of another hormone called glucagon. Glucagon production, as it relates to improving your body composition, is very important if your fitness goal is to lose excess body fat because it allows stored body fat to be released into the bloodstream to be burned by your muscles as energy. When the pancreas has to elevate its production of insulin while reducing its supply of glucagon, you are locking in your excess body fat. Therefore, too much simple sugar intake dramatically hinders the process of reducing stored body fat.

The consumption of sugar by Americans continues to rise year after year. So too does obesity. In my opinion, the correlation between increased sugar consumption and obesity is telling. When 16-20 percent of daily caloric intake is coming from sugar, Americans are not only locking in stored body fat, but also squeezing out the healthier, more supportive and nutrient-dense food choices. Sugar is the enemy of body fat reduction; and the enemy of a healthy, high energy lifestyle. Do your best to begin to understand what's in the food you are consuming and reduce those that contain more than a few grams of sugar.

When searching out food choices that include simple carbs, start by looking for obvious ingredients on food labels that actually use the word "sugar," e.g., brown sugar, sugar cane, and of course, simple sugar. Also, reduce your intake of foods that have any form of "syrup" in their ingredients, e.g., corn syrup, high fructose corn syrup, maple syrup and glucose syrup. And finally, look for those ingredients that end in "–ose" like sucrose, glucose, lactose and fructose. All of these ingredients are sugars and, if ingested, will spike your blood sugar and initiate the pancreas to produce insulin and essentially shut off glucagon production – the fat-release hormone.

If you find yourself in a situation where you are limited in your food choices (e.g., a breakfast or luncheon business meeting, traveling, dinner parties, etc.) and sugar seems to be the predominant choice, try to eat a protein with the sugar. Protein will help to slow down sugar's release into the bloodstream and reduce the insulin/glucagon effect.

Complex carbohydrates on the other hand, despite all the negative press they receive in some of the popular weight-loss books, are actually your body's preferred source of energy. When you consume the healthy complex carbs (the ones that have not been altered in a food laboratory), they are broken down into glucose molecules and used as fuel or stored in muscle and the liver as glycogen. When the body has an ample supply of glucose fuel and glycogen fuel storage, it can run efficiently. You then have the energy to function at your best and have provided the material that your body needs to reduce body fat and reach your health and fitness goals.

When you look for complex carbohydrate food choices to put into your body, seek out two subgroups of carbohydrates…starchy carbohydrates and fibrous carbohydrates. Starchy carbohydrates include food choices such as brown rice, baked and sweet potatoes, oatmeal, brown pastas and whole grains. Fibrous carbohydrates include asparagus, broccoli, cauliflower, onions, mushrooms, spinach and peppers and can also be found in most varieties of dark green leafy vegetables.

One more very important nugget of carbohydrate information to remember: Do your best to seek out the complex carbohydrates that have not been processed.

When shopping at the grocery store, stay away from the carbs that include the following words in their ingredients: bleached, enriched, processed or refined. These altered foods are void of critical nutrient value and will do very little to fuel and energize your body.

Bottom line - the goal in consuming carbohydrates should be to reduce or eliminate simple sugars and focus on complex carbohydrates, both the starchy and fibrous varieties, that have not been processed or refined.

At first, it may seem challenging as you begin to uncover the foods that contain sugar, eliminate them and seek out the more supportive carbohydrates. But once you get into the habit of eating the fibrous and starchy carbohydrates, it will become a way of life over time. I can promise you that after your initial efforts the payoff can be dramatic. Your energy level will soar. You will lose stubborn body fat. And your craving for sugar will completely dissipate.

Let me share the same simple steps with you that I share with my clients that will help you strive for your absolute physical best:

- Begin to gain an awareness of food labels and the "sugar" ingredients.

- Start to reduce or eliminate the simple sugars and the processed carbohydrates. Remember: If your goal is fat reduction, sugar is your worst enemy!

- Focus on making progress and forget about being perfect. You may slip up now and again. Just get back on track right away.

- Forgive yourself and just move on!

Champion Paul Ohashi's chapter on 'Strategies and Tips for Curing the Sugar-holic' will also be invaluable in helping you develop ways to reduce and/or eliminate sugar from your diet.

Remember that small changes over time will stack up on themselves…and eventually will bring you to a new destination of physical excellence!

Brian Calkins, B.A., ACE

513-325-0886
Brian.Calkins@thepowerofchampions.com
www.briancalkins.com

Strategies and Tips for Curing the Sugar-holic by Paul Ohashi

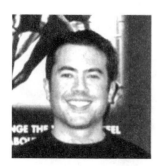

Champion Paul Ohashi of London, Ontario, Canada is Southwestern Ontario's elite body results specialist and fitness and health consultant. He currently trains at BodyWorx, London's premier private personal training studio.

Universal law of food consumption: If it is available, you will eat it. If it is not, you won't.

So there you are, confronted with the same dilemma once again: that candy bar is right in front of you. You feel hungry, and nothing would satisfy you more right now than smooth, buttery caramel enrobed in rich, velvety chocolate. Somewhere, very faintly in the distance of your mind, is a little voice reminding you that the treat is better left in its wrapper, that your energy level will sag thirty minutes after finishing it, that your blood sugar levels will spike and then plummet to new lows, that the subsequent hormonal events in your body will be counterproductive to your health, that insulin will make a three-hundred calorie deposit onto your hips, that you will regret eating that candy bar for well over an hour, and yet despite the honest reasoning of that little voice within you, you find some justification to grab that bar, tear into it and polish it off within a matter of minutes. There, that felt good, didn't it? But how do you really feel? Gradually, as the next few minutes go by, you notice things: guilt blossoms inside, you feel perky yet tired at the same time, and there is a bad taste in your mouth. You think, "If only I could have resisted eating that candy." And there, amidst the puddle of negative thoughts swelling in response to that candy bar, is that little voice again whispering just loud enough for you to hear "I told you so!"

Many of us have experienced a similar scenario at some point. Many of us go through it every day. If you do, you are not alone. I congratulate you for reading this chapter and taking the first step to conquering your sugar addiction. This could be one of the most important steps to your improved health. It takes a gutsy combination of physical effort, psychological willpower, and practical interventions to silence the incessant callings of sugar, but you would not still be reading if you did not have what it takes. The reward, I guarantee you, will feel wonderful. Below are ten easy steps you can follow that will dramatically improve your diet, but please remember they are only as effective as your action in implementing them. None of them are terribly difficult, but you will have to follow through consistently to emerge victorious. May the best in sugar-free health be yours.

Steps 1 - 3. The Practical

1. Do your grocery shopping on a full stomach and be in a good mood.

Two-thirds of your challenge can be won at the source by smart shopping. Not being hungry or upset when you shop means you will listen more to reason and less to your cravings. Supermarkets are filled with lots of wonderful food that will do wonderful things for you. They are filled with even more junk. Your primary objective is to prevent the junk from getting into your cupboards – to thwart the universal law.

2. Stick to the perimeter of your grocery store and only go into the aisles for staples you absolutely need.

Think about your grocery store and what is found along the perimeter: fruits and vegetables, lean meats, seafood, low-fat dairy, and whole-grain bakery products. This is all you need for a healthy diet. Unfortunately, too many of us spend too much time cruising the inner aisles of processed, refined food. Do yourself a favour: when you are shopping, start at the fruits and vegetables, and slowly make your way along the outside of the store. Only when you have almost filled your cart with good, wholesome food should you proceed into the inner aisles for those necessities on your shopping list. Even then, as you venture through the tempting towers of creams, cakes, and cookies, pick only those things you absolutely need.

3. Make pre-checkout observation a habit.

This step is *very* important and I do not want you to neglect it. Just before you are about to enter the checkout line, stop and take a good, long, honest look at everything in your cart or basket. Ask yourself this question about each item: "Is this product compatible with my health goals?" (I'm pretty sure you will know the answer.) The next step is then to simply take those products to which you answer "no" (of which there should not be many in your cart) and put them back on the shelf before returning to the checkout line.

Steps 4 - 6. The Physiological

4. Eat more frequently and ensure adequate protein and fiber at each meal.

This is extremely important: eat at least every three hours (5-7 small meals a day) and ensure adequate protein and fiber intake at each meal. The bare minimum is 5 grams of fiber and 10 grams of protein each meal. You may have to re-evaluate your supposedly healthy low-fat snacks. An apple needs more protein, yogurt lacks fiber, and a bagel falls short of both.

5. Use fruit as a sweet substitute. You'll avoid added fat while gaining nutrients, water, and fiber.

Granted, fruit contains sugar, and many fruits are high on the glycemic index. However, fruits are a natural, wholesome food, rich in vitamins, minerals, and antioxidants, high in water content, low in calories, and usually have some beneficial fiber. That sure beats anything refined and processed, so always have some fruit available.

6. Substitute longer-lasting, lower-calorie alternatives for the occasional sweet indulgence.

Choose hard candy over soft drinks, have a caramel candy instead of a glazed donut, or replace a chunk of chocolate with a chocolate candy. Simple choices, but they will put you on the path to success.

Steps 7 - 9. The Psychological

7. Before any meal, you must honestly answer one question. This is another *very* important point, but once you get used to it you will be much more in tune with your body and you will love yourself for it. Here is the question: "Am I eating this food to fulfill a physiological need for nourishment or am I fulfilling a psychological (and unnecessary) need?" Again, I think you can honestly answer this one yourself - if you listen to your body and not your tastebuds. Besides, if you are truly hungry, with an appetite for nourishment, all food - especially good, healthy food - will taste wonderful.

8. No craving is an all-or-nothing issue. By controlling the portion you eat, you win.

When you do occasionally find yourself in a battle of "I want to eat it" versus "I should not eat it," realize you do have power and use it. Acknowledge the presence of the food, accept that you want to have some, and know it isn't the best thing for you. Ask yourself the question in step #7. If you decide you are justified in having some, go ahead and eat just a tiny, little bit - and stop! Why? Because you just won. You just refused to let yourself lose. You could have eaten it all, but you didn't. Now put the food away and move on or seek a healthy alternative.

9. Gradually phase out foods that are high in sugar. Aim to eliminate one or two per month from your dietary repertoire.

Even eliminating one sugary food per month will greatly improve your diet if you are a regular consumer. Here are twelve possibilities you can easily live without: soft drinks, Pop-Tarts, cookies, chewy candies, jam, white bread, pancake syrup, alcoholic beverages, puddings, candy bars, cakes, muffins.

Step 10. The Test for Success

10. Pick one day this week and eliminate all sugars. Next week, do two consecutive days, the third week do three, and on the fourth week, do four consecutive days.

This easy task proves that, if you can survive even one day without sugars (and trust me, you will), the purpose of sugars in your diet is really not one of necessity. If you survive two days without sugar (and trust me, you can), ask yourself what purpose sugars had in your former diet. If you survive the four-day famine from sugar, you have begun teaching your body that it does not need sugar. If you have nourished yourself properly in those four days, you will notice a decreased craving for sweets, a more constant energy level, and a truly healthy appetite for wholesome foods.

Paul Ohashi, B.A., CPTN-CPT, CSCS

519-858-BODY
Paul.Ohashi@thepowerofchampions.com

Hydration by Kevin Gendron

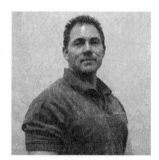

Champion Kevin Gendron of Shelton, Connecticut serves as Director of Sports Conditioning and is the founder of Better Athletic Development, a training facility specializing in injury prevention, speed development and programs such as Athlete's Edge-ucation™ and Performance Edge™.

What a beautiful day in the Caribbean Islands.

Soft, pink and white sands surround me, clear blue skies above me, a 95-degree sun, without the humidity, warming my lightly glistening body. A cool breeze off the leeward shore turns the pages of the novel I've been reading as a catamaran goes sailing by. How relaxing to just lie here and listen to the ocean crash against the shore away from the hustle and bustle of city life and work. Uh oh! Ow! Ow! Ow! I awake standing in my own bedroom with a calf cramp so painful it's like having my lower leg in a vice. "Gotta stretch it out!," I say to myself as I wonder how this painful dilemma could have happened.

Now I think I'm pretty fit, I exercise regularly, eat healthy and stretch often. My first thoughts were of the gym…boy, it's like playing desert hoops in there. I sweat so much it's like I just got out of the pool, fully clothed. One of the trainers at the gym says I need to drink more water. It couldn't be that simple. Or could it?

The Essential Nutrient

There are six categories of macronutrients that are essential for survival – vitamins, minerals, carbohydrates, proteins, fats and water. Of the six nutrients, water is the most essential in maintaining life (besides oxygen). We can survive for weeks without food, as magician David Blaine proved in his suspended glass box stunt consuming only water for 44 days, but only a few days without water.

Our body weight is approximately 70% water. The blood in our circulatory system is made up of 85% water. Although water contains no nutritional value, it is involved in almost every function of the body especially digestion, circulation, excretion and absorption. Protein and fat metabolism depend on water. Carbohydrates cannot be stored properly without it either.

Thermoregulation

Besides water's ability to cleanse your body by flushing toxins, lubricate your joints, assist with organ function and prevent your skin from drying out, one of the most important functions water provides is thermoregulation. The average normal body temperature is 98.6°F but may rise to as high as 104°F with intense exercise. Water in the form of sweat is your body's coolant through evaporation, your built-in air conditioner. As you exercise, your muscles generate heat, which is carried by the blood to the body's core. As core temperature rises, the heat is transported through capillaries near the skin's surface. Sweat glands release perspiration, which evaporates cooling the skin. Subdermal blood is transported back to the body's core cooling it.

Cooling will only take place if evaporation occurs. Water evaporation is a process requiring energy to change a liquid to a gas. Water as a gas contains more energy (heat) than its liquid state so as it evaporates it removes the heat from the skin's surface making you feel cooler.

On humid days, sweat evaporates more slowly because the atmosphere is already saturated with water vapor increasing the risk of heat-related illnesses, such as heat exhaustion, heat cramps and heat stroke. While your clothes may get soaked with sweat and you feel "cooler," no physical cooling actually takes place. Under extreme conditions and intense exercise, your body can produce approximately three liters of sweat equating to a 5-6 pound weight loss. If you don't replace that fluid during and after exercise, overheating and heat-related illnesses are likely to occur.

Maintaining hydration levels throughout the day by replacing water that is routinely lost through everyday activities, sweating and excretion is just as important as replenishing fluids following intense training and play. We need to consume water as part of our everyday regimen, not just during exercise.

The easiest way to determine your level of hydration is to weigh yourself prior to and following activity. If there's been more than a 2% loss in body weight, you will experience a decline in your performance primarily due to dehydration. Consistent fluid intake is the key to preventing this decline.

Overheating may also take place if the intensity of the exercise is so great that the working muscles compromise the circulatory system. While a certain portion of blood is used to regulate body temperature, large quantities of blood are still meeting the energy demands of the working muscles leaving an inadequate supply of blood for heat removal and ultimately a rise in core temperature.

Electrolytes

As your body loses water, the capacity of the blood to transport vital nutrients (glucose, fatty acids, oxygen) is lost. The blood's ability to remove the byproducts of metabolism (carbon dioxide and lactic acid) is also compromised. Coupled with this is a loss of electrolytes, sodium, potassium, chloride and magnesium, which are important for muscle contraction and relaxation. These minerals play a role in maintaining the body's fluid balance, assist with nutrient transport into the cells, tissue growth and repair and nerve impulse transmission.

This loss of fluid decreases blood volume which, in turn, increases the concentration of electrolytes in the blood, stimulating the thirst mechanism. Drinking pure water will satisfy the thirst mechanism, however, it may not provide for adequate rehydration. Water alone is not enough to support full fluid recovery when exercise lasts longer than one hour.

Research has found that adding carbohydrates along with sodium to water increases water's absorption rate from the small intestine into the bloodstream. A low carbohydrate concentration of between 6-8% appears to be ideal. This relates to between 14 and 19 grams of carbohydrate per 8 ounces of fluid. There are risks associated with a carbohydrate concentration above 8% which include diarrhea, nausea and cramping. More importantly, the additional sugars need to be digested, which in turn slows the absorption of fluid and is counterproductive to our goal of full rehydration. A carbohydrate concentration of 5% or less does not provide enough of an energy boost or increase the absorption rate.

Caffeine

Caffeine is a diuretic which aids in removing fluids from the body by stimulating urine production. In addition, if caffeine is present in your diet, it may have a slight ergogenic effect on performance if used sparingly; however, additional water intake is needed to replenish fluids lost from its use and rehydrate your body. Acceptable levels of caffeine are 3mg per kilogram of body weight or 1.5 mg of caffeine per pound of body weight. One cup of coffee contains approximately 120 mg of caffeine. One or two cups per day should be fine without increasing the risk of dehydration, diarrhea, dizziness, becoming jittery or throwing off your energy balance.

Carbonated Beverages

Avoid carbonated beverages and sodas (diet or regular) containing refined sugar. The added sugar will slow the absorption of fluid and the carbonation may make you feel bloated and full, decreasing your desire to drink. Furthermore, when you breathe your body is trying to expel the byproduct of the cardiovascular system in the form of carbon dioxide, the main ingredient found in all carbonated drinks.

Alcohol

Alcohol is even more of a diuretic than caffeine because it must be broken down by the liver and kidneys. The process consumes enormous amounts of water and explains why most people wake with cottonmouth after a night on the town. Cottonmouth is a sure sign of dehydration.

Rehydration

The National Athletic Trainers Association (NATA) has developed hydration guidelines based upon several years of research. The Association recommends that you consume 17 to 20 ounces of water or a sports drink two to three hours before any activity is performed. Ten to twenty minutes before starting your workout, 7 to 10 ounces of water or a sports drink should be consumed. Once activity has begun, NATA guidelines recommend drinking 7-10 ounces of water or sports drink every 10-15 minutes. Don't wait until you're thirsty. By then it's too late - the initial effects of dehydration on performance will have already started. Within two hours of activity, drink 20 ounces of water or a sports drink for every pound of body weight lost. This ensures proper fluid replacement. Recovery meals and proper post-workout hydration practices are vital to remaining at an optimal performance level.

It is recommended that, on average, you drink 55 percent of your body weight in fluid ounces per day. This will ensure your body stays fully hydrated and in peak performance mode throughout the day. For weight loss, up to 2/3 of an ounce of fluid per pound of body weight is recommended, or multiply your body weight by .65. For example, a 140 pound woman should drink approximately 77 ounces of fluid per day to remain fully hydrated and up to 91 ounces of fluid per day for weight loss. Additional rehydration options include consuming foods with high water content like salads, fresh fruits and vegetables throughout the day.

Getting back to my leg cramps, there are several theories that exist about the cause of muscle cramping, or sustained spasm. One theory states that during dehydration and fluid loss there is a decrease in blood volume therefore less blood flows to the muscles to deliver oxygen and nutrients causing spasm. A second theory is that an electrolyte imbalance is the culprit. Still another theory states that overly fatigued, overworked or under trained muscles may be more susceptible to cramping. Cold weather may also precipitate muscle cramps. Diabetics and individuals with circulatory or neurological disorders may be more susceptible to muscle cramps.

Remember that satisfying thirst doesn't necessarily mean you are satisfying your body's fluid needs. You must replenish fluids even though you're not thirsty. Remaining hydrated throughout the day will keep your body functioning at optimal levels both at work and at play and will dramatically improve your chances of reaching your health and fitness goals.

Kevin Gendron, MS, CSCS

Better Athletic Development
33 Hull Street, Suite 3
Shelton, CT 06484
203-924-2230
Kevin.Gendron@thepowerofchampions.com
www.betterathletes.net

The Low Carb Myth by Brad Schoenfeld

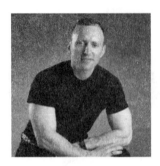

Champion Brad Schoenfeld of Scarsdale, New York has a new book, *The Look Great Naked Diet* (Avery Penguin Putnam), which explains his breakthrough program for optimizing a person's genetic shape and reducing body fat to levels previously thought impossible.

Scan the current crop of bestsellers and you'll notice a recurring theme: diet books.

Not just any diet books, mind you, but ketogenic (i.e., low carb) diet books. *Sugarbusters*, *Protein Power*, *The Carbohydrate Addict's Diet*…the list goes on and on. Although these types of diets have been used for many years in the treatment of epilepsy, it wasn't until Dr. Robert Atkins published his book, *Dr. Atkins' Diet Revolution*, that they really came into the mainstream. Today, low carb is a phenomenon, with millions of devoted followers worldwide.

If past experience is any indication, chances are good that you are tempted to try a low carb diet…or perhaps you're even counting carbs as we speak. Heck, hardly a day goes by where a client doesn't ask me about the subject. To be sure, a great deal of controversy exists about these diets and questions remain as to their efficacy. Nutritionists tend to be polarized on the subject. On one side are the ketogenic proponents who claim that eliminating dietary carbohydrate is the key to achieving a lean body; on the other side are those who claim that ketogenic diets are a one-way ticket to liver failure, renal dysfunction and a plethora of other ailments. So where does the truth lie? The answer is somewhere in between.

Although every book on low-carb dieting has a slightly different wrinkle, they all share the same focus - inducing ketosis. Ketosis is a compensated state where the body shifts from using carbohydrates (glucose) to ketones—a byproduct of the incomplete breakdown of fatty acids—for energy. Proponents of these diets profess that, by regulating insulin function and shifting the body into a "fat-burning mode," ketosis optimizes weight loss while helping to preserve lean muscle tissue—quite a lofty claim indeed.

The truth is, however, the research supporting these contentions is scant, at best. Without question, ketogenic diets help to stabilize insulin levels. Insulin is a storage hormone. While its primary purpose is to neutralize blood sugar, it also is responsible for shuttling fat into adipocytes (fat cells). When carbohydrates are ingested, the pancreas secretes insulin to clear blood sugar from the circulatory system. Depending on the quantities and types of carbs consumed, insulin levels can fluctuate wildly, heightening the possibility of fat storage.

Making matters worse, many people are insulin resistant—as much as a quarter of the population by some estimates. In fact, it is postulated that anyone who is clinically obese (i.e., more than 20 percent over his or her ideal body weight) has at least some degree of insulin resistance. This condition prevents glucose from entering target cells, resulting in the conversion of carbohydrate to fat (through a process called lipogenesis). A vicious cycle is created, whereby fat storage is increased and insulin resistance is heightened even further. Eventually, this can lead to the onset of non-insulin dependent diabetes (NIDD)—a serious disease that causes blindness, stroke and even death.

However, although ketogenic diets are quite effective at regulating blood sugar, by no means are they necessary to combat insulin resistance. For the great majority of people, simply cutting back carb intake to about 40 percent of total calories is sufficient to accomplish this task.[39, 40] Even in extreme cases, a drastic reduction in carbohydrates rarely is needed to stabilize insulin levels.

Furthermore, there is little evidence that inducing a state of ketosis actually helps to accelerate fat loss and/or preserve muscle. While the rationale behind a "fat-burning mode" sounds great in theory, it simply doesn't translate into practice.[41] Studies have shown that it's the total energy intake, rather than the composition of macronutrients, that is the major determinant in the loss of body fat.[42, 43] This is consistent with the first law of thermodynamics: If you expend more calories than you consume, you'll lose weight. Provided there is a caloric deficit, the body seems to adjust its substrate utilization, burning similar amounts of fat regardless of dietary nutritional composition. Champion Kelly Huggins offers more insight into the law of thermodynamics in his chapter, 'Burn Fat by Eating More!'

But what about the testimonials from people claiming to lose as much as fifteen pounds in the first two weeks of dieting? Well, much of this reduction is due to a loss of fluids—not body fat.[44] You see, carbs have a propensity to attract water in the body (each gram of stored carbohydrate attracts about three times its weight in water). Hence, when carbs are eliminated from the diet, diuresis is encouraged causing the kidneys to excrete water. But while this can provide a psychological boost in the early stages of dieting, the fervor is relatively short-lived. As soon as the diet is discontinued and carbs are reintroduced into your system, all of the water weight returns—an outcome that can be extremely disheartening and can even lead to post-diet depression.

In truth, the real "magic" behind ketogenic diets is their effect on appetite suppression; when carbs are restricted, food cravings tend to subside. Although the exact mechanism for this is unclear, it is theorized that increased secretions of satiety hormones play an integral role in the process. The hormones cholecystokinin (CCK) and glucagon, in particular, are believed to quell hunger sensations, reducing the urge to eat.[45]

Additionally, due to a limited number of food choices, there is less pleasure associated with eating low-carb meals. With reduced variety, food becomes mundane, even boring. After several weeks of subsisting on nothing but protein and fat, most people never want to look at another piece of steak or cheese again! The net result: a diminished caloric intake. This is the philosophy behind Atkins' assertion that you can eat as much as you want on his diet; he knows that you won't!

On the other hand, it is important to note that ketogenic diets aren't a one-way ticket to the emergency ward either. The doom-and-gloom warnings that these diets pose severe health risks are, in the very least, seriously overstated. No peer-reviewed studies have shown that restricting carbohydrate intake is detrimental to liver or kidney function (although there is an increased tendency toward the development of kidney stones). Similarly, little evidence exists that cardiovascular risk factors are negatively impacted by low carb diets. This is because the complications from saturated fat consumption are cumulative, not immediate. It takes many years for symptoms to manifest. Thus, even though there is a large amount of saturated fat intake associated with low-carb eating, it is highly unlikely that this can cause any detrimental effects in the short-term. In fact, most people who are obese actually see a positive impact on their lipid profiles simply due to losing weight.[46, 47]

In the final analysis, ketogenic diets aren't the nutritional panacea touted by some, nor are they the Pandora's Box claimed by others. The problem with these diets, as with any other type of diet, is that they don't teach you proper eating habits.[48] Diets are short-term solutions to a long-term problem—which is why 90 percent of all dieters regain their weight after one year.

So what's the take home message here? Balance! The key to promoting long-term, sustainable weight management is to develop a sound nutritional strategy that becomes a way of life. Nutrition is much more complex than simply cutting carbs (or cutting fat for that matter) from your diet. You need to customize a dietary regimen that balances caloric intake with caloric expenditure, focusing on both amounts and the kinds of nutrients that you consume. (For example, white bread is not metabolized in the same way as multi-grain bread and margarine does not have the same effect on your body as flaxseed oil!) I've worked with people from all walks of life who, by applying the aforementioned principles, have seen the amazing long-term transformations that have taken place when proper protocols are followed. If they can do it, so can you!

Brad Schoenfeld, CSCS

Brad.Schoenfeld@thepowerofchampions.com
www.lookgreatnaked.com

Creatine? by John Spencer Ellis

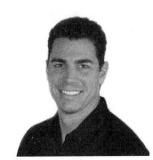

Champion John Spencer Ellis of Rancho Santa Margarita, California is the president of NESTA (National Endurance & Sports Trainers Association). He holds 15 health, fitness and medical certifications. In addition, he has a 2nd degree black belt in kung fu and has completed the Ironman triathlon.

Creatine is a hot topic today for almost any weightlifter as well as anyone involved in any sport consisting of explosive short bursts of energy.

These would include a thirty-second play in football, basketball, boxing, etc. The benefits of creatine usage for some lifters are so fantastic that it becomes somewhat mystical for newcomers. The purpose of this chapter is to explain the "mechanics" of creatine in a non-technical way, to be a guideline for its use, and to be a reference point. Lately, the information about creatine has been distorted, exaggerated, and misunderstood. Let's completely understand this unique enhancement tool.

Creatine (usually in the form of creatine monohydrate) is a supplement taken to enhance anaerobic (strength and/or power) performance. Creatine monohydrate (CM) is a white, odorless crystalline powder, clear and colorless in solution. Creatine is nontoxic, even in large amounts.

CM is a popular supplement that serves as an energy reserve in muscle cells. Once it enters muscle cells, creatine monohydrate becomes creatine phosphate (CP). Muscular contraction is powered by the breakdown of ATP (adenosine triphosphate) to ADP (adenosine diphosphate). When ATP is broken down, CP in the muscle phosphorilates (donates a phosphate group to) ADP changing it back to ATP so that further energy reactions can occur. CM is a precursor to creatine phosphate. By supplementing with CM, CP levels in muscle are maximized and maintained elevated so that more muscular work can occur, since there are greater energy reserves to use.

CM also helps with resistance training by loading the muscle with creatine rich fluid. The term "cell volumization" refers to the increased volume of fluid and cellular materials caused by creatine supplementation. When creatine enters the cell, it brings fluid into the cell with it. This higher level of fluid and cellular materials allow for greater leverage and requires the muscle to move less and lift more weight. While this may seem somewhat trivial, some researchers today think that one of the stimulating factors of steroid use is cell volumization due to increased intracellular (inside the cell) water retention. Anabolic steroids may actually work in part because of cellular fluid retention in the muscles. The swelling action and the related stretching of the cells may in and of itself cause a reaction, which stimulates the muscle cells to grow. So in that respect creatine might be as good as steroids without the many side effects that may be caused by steroid use. Many people report increasing their lean muscle mass between 6 to 14 lbs. while using CM.

Some people report symptoms including headaches, clenched teeth, and the sound of blood rushing in their ears while using CM. These symptoms are the same as experienced with high blood pressure. Creatine's effects on blood pressure are still being researched. Since it has the effect of increasing fluid concentration in muscle, it might increase blood pressure in the same way high levels of sodium do. Although sodium tends to increase blood pressure by increasing serum or blood volume via its hydrophilic (water loving) nature, it also may increase intracellular fluid depending on the sodium concentration. The effects of creatine on blood pressure have not been established or refuted.

In addition, one other symptom reported is stomach cramps. Reducing the intake of CM saw a reduction in the severity of the cramps. The most common problem seen with creatine use, however, is muscle cramping. Many athletes, especially football players, report increased hamstring cramps and pulls. Because creatine carries extra-cellular fluid into the cell, it may cause dehydration believed to cause muscle pulls and cramps. These can be avoided by maintaining adequate hydration status. Champion Kevin Gendron's chapter, 'Hydration,' is a very useful resource for determining fluid intake and which sources are the most effective.

Creatine seems to be well studied in scientific research. Scientific evidence supporting creatine is there, but while some very good results have been reported, such as a 20 lb. body weight gain in 6 weeks and strength increases, others have reported no significant gains whatsoever while taking the supplement. The reason for this great disparity is believed to be the many different types and brands of creatine available in the market today. CM is available in effervescent form, liquid, tablets, and even as a candy. The only type that has clinical trials backing up its effectiveness is the regular powder form. The main drawback of creatine usage is its price.

The most effective type is in capsule form which also contains a matrix of Kreb's cycle intermediaries (aspartates and succinates) chelated with critical electrolytes to amplify cellular uptake and utilization of creatine by a factor which is calculated to be as high as 300%. Aspartates promote decreased ammonia production and increased ammonia removal thus reducing ammonia toxicity. Succinates promote calcium homeostasis necessary for non-catabolic muscle metabolism and maximum force of contraction. Electrolytes restore depleted muscle cell stores of potassium, magnesium and calcium commonly resulting from physical exercise. This type of superior absorption and metabolism eliminates the loading and maintenance doses initially believed to be necessary. This results in elimination of potential stomach upset and greatly reduced creatine loss due to gut breakdown and urinary excretion. According to Lucho Crisalle RD, NESTA's director of nutrition, as of the date of this release, Cell Charge by Bio Nutritional Research Group is the only creatine in the market designed with the Kreb's cycle matrix mentioned above.

If you take creatine monohydrate and don't notice any results in about 2 weeks, it's a good bet that you have chosen a low quality supplement. Once you plateau, your muscle cells will probably be saturated with creatine and since the body loses about 1-2% creatine a day you should be able to get away with cycling on and off creatine to lengthen your results. Once you stop creatine supplementation and your body clears it 100% (6 to 8 weeks), you will most likely have retained a portion of the muscle and strength gained. Of course the gains in mental ability and tendon/skeletal strength increase resulting from these heavier workouts will remain.

Pharmacology - Creatine occurs in highest concentrations in skeletal muscle, followed by cardiac and smooth muscle, brain, kidney and spermatozoa. Strenuous exercise rapidly uses up cellular reserves of CP to replace ATP, the only chemical that powers muscle contraction and relaxation.

Proper use - Of course, first read the label and any additional leaflets that come with your brand of creatine monohydrate.

Although initially it was recommended to go through a loading phase of 20 to 30 grams daily for five to six days, to be followed by 3 to 5 grams daily for four to six weeks, it is now recommended that you take creatine after exercise with a glucose (NOT fructose) load. There is a new thought process in this regard. Don't mix creatine with citrus juice. Orange, grapefruit, cranberry, in fact, most fruit juices have been most recently found to neutralize the activity of creatine monohydrate. The reason is that the waste product creatinine develops. Many of you who use CM now may put creatine on your tongue and drink it down with grapefruit juice. If you have taken creatine this way in the past, stop it now! You are not getting creatine, you're getting waste product. This is because of the fructose in the above-named juices. Pharmaceutical grade glucose or even dextrose is preferred as these do cause an increase in insulin secretion, which in turn will shuttle the CM into the cell along with fluid, etc. It is recommended to drink lots of water while on creatine.

The University of Florida conducted a study where three groups were randomly selected to either:

- Take 5g five times per day CM for a five day "loading phase," and six weeks worth of placebo.
- A placebo-loading phase with six weeks worth of CM.
- A placebo-loading phase and six-week period (control group).

A muscle biopsy was done at the end of the study and found that both groups that took creatine had the same amount of creatine in muscle cells. This proved that it is not necessary to "load."

Note: The use of caffeine is discouraged while on creatine; creatine makes your muscles hold water while caffeine will do the opposite, thereby reducing the effects of the creatine intake. There is also thought to be an allosteric interaction between caffeine and CM.

Be sure to drink a full eight-ounce glass of good water 8 times a day. Creatine pulls water from other parts of the body to perform its work in expanding muscle cells. You need 1 ounce of water for every 30 calories you consume.

You should be aware that creatine, because the FDA categorizes it as a food supplement, isn't subject to the same stringent manufacturing requirements as medications. This means that the amount and quality of creatine that you purchase may vary from one company to another or even between batches from the same company.

John Spencer Ellis, B.S., MBA, Ed.D.

29832 Avenida de las Banderas
Rancho Santa Margarita, CA 92688
949-589-9166
JohnSpencer.Ellis@thepowerofchampions.com
www.NestaCertified.com

SECTION SEVEN
Perform Like a Champion

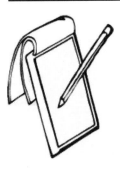

Notes from Phil

It's all abut performance. Of course when it comes to athletes, the performance is the game. While your fitness program helps you improve function in virtually every area of endeavor, specialized training can help you find greater reward on the tennis court . . .or yes, even the golf course!

Golf and tennis both provide analogies for real-life movement. You use your entire body, you incorporate balance, muscle control, coordination, and focus. It's no wonder these two sports have found widespread popularity not only among elite professionals, but among weekend warriors and novices alike.

Our Champions have come to understand both the athlete's physical needs and psyche and, in this section, Champion Noel Lyons offers some practical advice for anyone who finds pleasure, frustration, or a combination of the two in swinging a golf club. Noel teaches you to "get in shape to play your sport," which is a far cry from the oft-made mistake of believing that playing your sport gets you in shape. Champion Gina Piazza expands on the idea of fitness to benefit the golfer by helping you identify "the missing link." Finally, Champion Robert Selders shares the crucial elements of an effective and safe tennis fitness program.

Whatever your sport or athletic preference, you'll find wisdom among the Champions that will lead to greater prowess and performance.

Fitness Lessons for Optimal Golf... and for Optimal Living by Noel Lyons

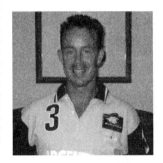

Champion Noel Lyons of Marbella, Spain is the Med Golf Fitness Consultant. With his coaching and support, David Steele was able to break the European Golf Marathon record with 774 holes in 24 hours (43 rounds averaging 76 per round)!

Golf – Not Just a Sport - More a Way of Life

Golf is fast becoming the world's most popular sport with as many as 60 million participants worldwide. As a Personal Trainer on the Costa del Sol/Costa del Golf (with the highest density of golf courses on the European continent), I work with numerous golfers who are passionate about their sport. So let me share with you the secret of playing golf well ......well into your golden years!

Get in shape to play your sport. Don't play your sport to get in shape.

Most club golfers think they get "fit" by playing golf. Unfortunately, this is not the case. Most players do not walk the course at a sufficient pace to improve their aerobic fitness.

Furthermore, most club golfers step onto the first tee, fling their club around themselves 3-4 times as a warm up, and then fire their first shot at 85 to 100 mph. No wonder they get hurt!

The more diligent might practise their swing for hours, with the intention of working on their game. However, if your musculoskeletal system isn't conditioned for the extra strain, over-practising a swing can do more harm than good!

Sharing the Secret – Better Golf, Better Living

You see, unfortunately "playing" and "practising" golf is not enough. You must treat your game and body like the golf pros do. You need to add a structured and regular 'golf-specific' exercise programme to your routine.

By understanding which specific exercises can improve your golf game, you will also start to understand which exercises are important for your general health and fitness, as well as for those slowing-down, age-related declines in the body. In other words, the very same exercises that contribute to better golf also contribute to a better quality of life, particularly as you age.

Exercise – How It Can Improve Your Golf Game

- Increases your driving power
- Decreases your injury potential
- Increases your satisfaction with the game (better golf, lower scores)
- Allows you to play without feeling fatigued and to stay focused
- Allows you to play more often (as you recover quicker from playing)
- Keeps you playing well into your golden years

Exercise - How It Can Improve Your Overall Health and Vitality (provided you walk the course!)

- Walking 18 holes = 3+ miles, particularly if you don't hit the ball straight every time!
- Helps maintain your lean muscle mass and basal metabolic rate
- The balance and coordination involved keeps you agile
- Wards off degenerative diseases and maintains functional independence
- Decreases anxiety and tension, which helps regulate blood pressure
- Reduces total cholesterol and increases the good high density lipoprotein cholesterol (HDL)
- Valuable relaxation time close to nature for renewed energy and vitality
- Social atmosphere (playing in groups of 2, 3 or 4 plus tournament play)

Quite simply exercise can add years to your golfing life, and life to your golfing years!

The Role of Exercise in the Modern Game of Golf

There is perhaps no single action in sport that requires more overall muscular strength, joint flexibility, and movement coordination than a perfectly executed golf swing. As a result, today's top young players are leaner, more muscular, and more flexible than the generation of golfers before them.

Muscle Suppleness

In my view, this is perhaps the most important requirement. I watch many "seniors" on the coast practise their swing through a limited range of movement.

Individual restrictions in your body can prevent you from doing what the teacher, video or golf magazine says you must if you want to improve your game. What the pro sees as a swing fault is often only the manifestation of how you attempt to compensate for a limitation. In addition, injuries can keep golfers off the course for long periods and eventually force retirement from the game.

Stretching is vitally important to ensure that your body can move through the range of motion required in the golf swing without causing excessive stress on the muscles or joints. Tight muscles lead to shorter drives, so you must increase your flexibility if you want to play — and live — comfortably. Smooth, coordinated movements lead to consistency in your swing.

What's more, arthritis is the major affliction for individuals 50 years of age and older. Recent research suggests that many incidences could be prevented if people took time to stretch. Simply hitting balls at the driving range won't increase your mobility or loosen your tight muscles. You need a daily stretching and mobility routine to find comfort on the golf course — and afterward.

Here's one simple mobility exercise - kneel on both knees, with your hands resting on the back of your hips. Now pass your club through the gap between your back and your elbows. Your knees should be shoulder width apart or just fractionally inside. Your posture is the same as it would be if you were addressing a shot.

Now turn your shoulders as much as you can to the right or as you would normally do on your backswing. When doing this let your left hip turn to the right with your turn. Your knees should not move and expect some resistance down your left hand side. Repeat 12 times both sides. This drill can add power to your backswing.

Muscle Strength and Endurance

In golf, it is important to maintain your spine angle for a consistent swing. This means you remain bent or tilted at the hips. This requires sufficient strength and flexibility in your hamstrings, abdominals and lower back. If any of these are weak or tight, you will struggle. The result is often off-centre hits, less distance, errant shots, and post-golf soreness in the back! Champion Katie Mital's chapter, 'My Aching Back,' gives practical advice for preventing low back pain and how to deal with it when it flares up.

To strengthen your hamstrings, try lunges. Take a big step forward and drop your body weight onto the front leg and let the back leg knee almost touch the ground (hips and knees should be at a 90 degree angle). Keeping your body upright, return to the starting position. Repeat 12 times on each leg. For a more detailed description of lunges and associated exercises, check out Champion Darrell Morris' chapter, 'Reducing and Shaping Your Hips and Thighs.'

Optimal golf also demands adequate strength in your shoulders and arms, as these connect your golf club with your body's "core." By strength-training 2-3 times a week, you will also help combat age-related loss of muscle mass and increase your bone mineral density.

Muscle Balance and Agility

The golf swing is a motion that involves all parts of your body. Force is transferred from the ankles, to the legs, to the back, to the shoulders and through the wrists. The smoother the transfer of force, the better. Hence, it is important to build "whole-body" exercises into your programme, often on unstable surfaces, to encourage "movement efficiency" and coordinated actions between muscle groups.

Not only will this add a level of consistency to your game, balance and agility is key in later life to prevent falls and similar accidents.

Cardiovascular Fitness - Keeping Body Fat Levels Down

Without a cardio component in a golfer's training routine, fatigue often sets in and limits the quality practise time required to make lasting changes in the golf swing. Concentration levels also drop toward the end of a game.

Tired, unfit golfers practise faulty movement patterns that can take over for correct golf techniques. These improper movement patterns practised when you are tired may influence your swing when you are fresh and rested.

The best thing you can do for your health is to keep any excess weight off. For a golfer, a potbelly will also affect the centre of the swing. Not convinced? Simply look at the top ten golfers in your country. All have narrow hips, a flat stomach, wide shoulders and a strong back. Such conditioning is all geared toward maximising distance and consistency in their drive.

Get In Shape for Golf! Get In Shape for Life!

Without regular exercise a golfer finds their strength, mobility and agility, so vital to the game, gradually diminish with age. By improving strength, mobility, coordination and aerobic fitness, you can expect to have better control over your body across 18 holes, thus optimizing swing mechanics and accuracy, resulting in fewer "miss-hits" and lower scores.

So through combining golf practise with golf-specific conditioning exercises, I guarantee not only will you look and feel years younger... you'll also have a good chance to beat some of the younger players you might get paired with!

Noel Lyons, MSc, B.A., ACSM

Noel.Lyons@thepowerofchampions.com
www.pureproactivity.com

Golf Conditioning by Gina M. Piazza

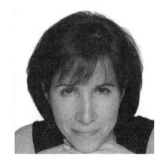

Champion Gina M. Piazza of Saddle River, New Jersey is the president of gmp fitness, LLC, creator of two award winning programs, FIT TO BREAK PAR and 9 HOLE GOLF FITNESS®, has appeared on the Golf Channel and featured in many publications including *Golf, Golf Digest, Senior Golfer, PGA Magazine, Golf For Women* among others.

Golf is one of the fastest growing sports.

The pursuit of excellence, the attempt to be perfect and consistent in each and every round occupies amateur and professional players alike. Some play for relaxation, others play for exercise and many play for business entertainment.

The common goal...great shots and lower scores. To do this, golfers will spend countless hours at the driving range, take lesson upon lesson and invest thousands of dollars in training aids only to be frustrated by a round of golf filled with poor hits, bogeys, chronic injuries, fatigue and pain.

Why? Because the most important lesson and training aid has been overlooked and left out.

The missing link...A healthy, physically fit body.

A Healthy Body

The golf swing engages your entire body. Every time you swing the club, all your bones, joints and muscles twist and turn. Golfers are constantly bending over to pick up balls and putt in a bent over stance. Couple this with the repetitive motion of the golf swing, fatigue that comes from a round of golf, as well as incorrect body mechanics. Now add the fact that many golfers bring a previous injury to the game. Finally, add muscle imbalance, poor posture and inflexibility that can exacerbate the problem. What do you get? "High Risk Injury Potential."

Golf Injuries

Muscle tears, tendonitis and ligament strains are some of the injuries that are prevalent among golfers. These injuries tend to occur more frequently to the upper back and neck, the lower back, the rotator cuff, the elbow ("golfer's elbow") and the wrist. Many of the injuries golfers incur are caused by the repetitive motion of the golf swing. Moreover, many golfers bring a previous injury to the game. Continued play with an existing injury creates stress on other muscles and may develop a secondary injury.

Do you want to be a better golfer, avoid injuries and pain? Then be proactive.

Are you currently playing with a pre-existing injury? If so, you'll want to seek professional help. A professional can perform an evaluation, diagnosis, treatment, prevention and rehabilitation of golf injuries, and offer preventative swing advice. If you are lucky enough to be injury free, then it's time to prepare your body for a round of golf.

Golf Conditioning

Being able to hit consistent shots not only depends on understanding how to swing the golf club, but also relies on your body's ability to do so. Your physically fit body is an essential component to the success of the golf swing. Many golfers believe that a regular exercise program is not necessary in order to improve their individual performance. This misconception has plagued golfers for years with pain and discomfort.

Golf is an athletic sport that requires a physically fit body. What elements make up a physically fit body?

- Centered posture - the critical building block for movement efficiency
- Good balance - establishes a stable stance for tempo and swing consistency
- Core stability - protects the spine for movement during the golf swing
- Overall flexibility - enhances your ability to turn and generate faster club head speed
- Increased strength - creates more power and club control

When getting ready to embark on a golf-specific program make sure to include functional fitness tools. What kind of equipment do you need?

- Stability Ball - promotes better balance, improved posture and increased flexibility
- Medicine Ball - encourages greater coordination, stamina and strength
- Resistance Cords - reinforce the patterns of the golf swing and help strengthen your muscles
- Foam Rollers and Balance Discs/Boards - improve balance, especially when performing the golf swing on these unstable exercise devices

One of the most popular fitness tools is the stability ball. Did you know that many professional golfers utilize the stability ball as part of their conditioning program? This all-encompassing exercise device works more than one muscle group at the same time, plus conditioning with the ball will:

- Heighten postural awareness
- Increase flexibility
- Develop strength
- Reinforce stabilization
- Improve balance

Here's an example of a conditioning move using the stability ball to get you started.

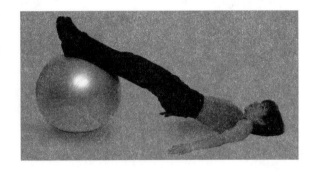

Level 1 - Lie on the floor on your back with the ball under the bend of your knees. Place your hands on the floor at your sides. Tighten and lift your buttocks and hips off the floor. Return to the starting position and repeat.

Level 2 - As you begin to feel balanced and comfortable with this exercise, position the ball under your calves and repeat as above.

There are many variations that you can do to make the exercise more challenging. For example, try crossing your arms over your chest and perform the same move. This will encourage trunk stabilization (rather than relying on the hands for control) as you lift your buttocks off the floor.

What About Conditioning on the Course?

Did you know that most amateur golfers will show up at the course only minutes before their tee time without doing a proper warm up? If your body is tight, it will definitely cause mechanical problems in the swing and put you at risk for injury.

To hit good golf shots, your muscles must be properly prepared. Stretching is a key element in many professional golfers' pre-game routines. Proper conditioning should consist of moves to warm up your body, increase blood circulation and lengthen your muscles. A flexible and limber body will increase range of motion in your swing, add control and power, create a relaxed mental state, reduce the likelihood of injury and enhance your overall performance. To help prevent injury and improve your swing mechanics, take a few minutes to condition your body before and during play.

Here's an example of a conditioning move to get you ready for the first tee. Pictured on page 204.

Hold a club just outside shoulder width. Place your feet hip width apart. Lower your body bending at your knees and hips (no further than 90°) and at the same time lift the club above your head. Then straighten your legs and lower your arms back down to the starting position. Perform this move 15 times. Move slowly and in a controlled manner.

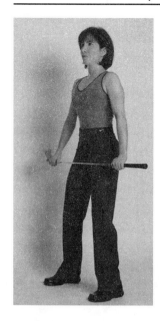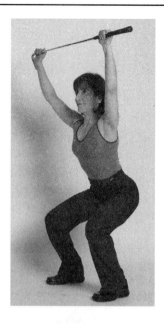

And Finally...Follow the Essential Wellness Tips

In addition to on-course stretching, there are several essential wellness tips that golfers should follow on the course. These include skin and lip protection, eye protection, proper hydration, sound nutrition and proper foot attire.

Skin and Lip Protection
Use a sunscreen that is proven effective against both UVA and UVB rays. By using a little common sense and good quality products, you may reduce your chances of skin and lip damage.

Eye Protection
Shield your eyes with UV-blocking sunglasses. The right pair of sunglasses is the best defense and best way to protect your eyes in either a sunny or cloudy environment.

Proper Hydration
Golfers must drink water while on the course. Don't wait until you are thirsty to drink. Drinking water is essential for concentration and muscle coordination, both necessary for an effective golf swing.

Sound Nutrition
Your body will perform better when properly fueled with the right diet. Nutritious foods will give you the leverage you need to improve concentration, have more stamina and feel better.

Proper Foot Attire
A good pair of golf shoes should not make your feet uncomfortable during or at the end of a round of golf. Problems with the feet can inhibit tempo and balance and transfer further problems to the spine and the rest of the body. If pain persists, speak to your healthcare practitioner. He or she can diagnose and treat any problems.

Summing It Up

Your swing is only as good as your physical abilities will allow. If you're looking for game improvement, lower scores and to feel great playing golf, get started today. To develop a solid golf game, a total approach needs to be taken and you must be willing to commit.

You may want to consider investing in a couple of golf fitness books and/or videos. These are excellent reference tools for exercise design. Or consider hiring a certified personal trainer on a consulting basis to help design a golf-specific workout for you and update it periodically. These professionals can motivate you, make certain you are doing the exercises properly and help you achieve your goals. To find a trainer in your area go to www.thepowerofchampions.com.

Whatever you decide, be a stroke ahead of your golf game. By incorporating conditioning exercises and following the on-course wellness tips, you will be on your way to a better round of golf, further reducing the chance of injury and, most of all, enjoying a fulfilling and fun game of golf.

Stay healthy and enjoy your next round of golf!

Gina M. Piazza, B.S., AAHFRP

gmp fitness, LLC
Saddle River, NJ 07458
1-888-467-3488
Gina.Piazza@thepowerofchampions.com
www.gmpfitness.com

Tennis Fitness, Anyone? by Robert L. Selders, Jr.

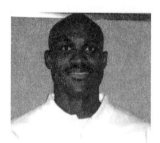

Robert L. Selders, Jr. of Rowlett, Texas is a Sports Performance Specialist at Velocity Sports Performance and conducts fitness training sessions at Your Personal Trainer Fitness Studio. He is currently pursuing a Master's degree in Exercise Science and Health Promotion.

Many consider tennis to be the perfect lifetime sport: you can get an intense workout with regular rest periods, compete at any skill level and age for as long as you wish, and in the process, improve your overall health and quality of life.

Obtaining lessons from a qualified tennis professional and playing on a consistent basis will allow you to make considerable progress in your tennis game. However, in order to truly enjoy tennis and be competitive, not only must you possess the knowledge and skill to play, but your body must also be physically capable of handling the stresses that accompany the sport. Preparing your body in this manner will make you less susceptible to those nagging injuries that can keep you sidelined.

An effective tennis fitness program contains several components that are designed to minimize injury potential while improving overall strength and conditioning levels for tennis. The basic components should include elements of *F*lexibility, *A*gility, *S*trength, and *T*ennis-specific mental preparedness. Participating in a training program that utilizes components of the *F.A.S.T.* approach will help ensure optimal performance on the court. As with any sports or fitness training program, it is advisable to consult with your physician before starting a sports or fitness training program.

Your tennis fitness program should be tailored to meet your individual needs in order to maximize the training effect while minimizing injury potential. The following will briefly examine each element of the *F.A.S.T.* approach.

Flexibility. Flexibility is the degree to which soft tissues (muscles, tendons, and connective tissue) extend to allow full range of motion (ROM) about a particular body joint. The two primary types of flexibility are static and dynamic flexibility. Static flexibility refers to the total ROM about a joint during passive movement while dynamic flexibility is the available ROM during active movement.

Tennis is a sport that requires participants to move in multiple planes with relatively wide ranges of motion. Players must have the ability to generate high degrees of force from any number of body positions, e.g., returning a wide shot, serving, extending for a drop shot, etc. Having adequate strength levels throughout each joint's full range of motion will enhance performance and minimize injury potential.

Before playing tennis, you should always warm up to help prepare your body to better respond to the subsequent stresses and prevent injury. Current research suggests using dynamic flexibility exercises (controlled movements that are identical to the activity to be performed) to stimulate the proper neuromuscular pathways and prime the body for more efficient movement. Since static flexibility exercises initiate a relaxation response in muscles, they should be performed during the cool down phase or after you play. For example, prior to a match you should take about 5 minutes and perform light cardio work, e.g., a series of jumping jacks, light jogging, or calisthenics, to increase your heart rate and raise your body's core temperature. Afterwards, you should spend another 5-10 minutes performing dynamic flexibility movements. Exercises like arm circles, multi-planar lunges, lateral shuffles, swinging your racquet, trunk twists, or any other tennis-specific movement will certainly do the trick.

Agility. Agility can be defined as possessing the physical capability to decelerate, stabilize, and accelerate to either change direction or speed of movement, while maintaining good posture, balance, and body control. In order to perform even the most basic tennis strokes, great footwork is required to move from the ready stance into the proper position for stroke execution. Being more agile allows you to accomplish this by developing the ability to control your center of gravity. When combined with speed and quick reaction time, agility will allow you to increase your movement range to close on the ball faster and position yourself to consistently hit more solid and powerful ground strokes. There are many drills and training aids, e.g., agility ladder, reaction balls, etc., that can be used to improve agility. Agility training should not be done when your body is in a fatigued state…remember, movement quality, and not quantity, is the primary goal.

Strength. Tennis is an intrinsically ballistic sport that exposes your body to high levels of stress. The goal of a tennis-specific strength training program should be to develop muscular and speed endurance, rotational power, and joint stability. Increasing muscular strength (not bulk) through resistance training will help your body to better absorb and distribute the forces to reduce injury potential in joints and connective tissue. Since muscle mass is not the primary goal, you should use higher repetitions with moderate resistance levels to build muscular endurance. Build cardiovascular and speed endurance using proper work to rest ratios to help give you that extra stamina to outlast your opponents. You can add more pace to your stroke by developing rotational power with multi-planar medicine ball throws, cable movements, and resistance bands. Joint stabilization is critical to optimal performance; without it, you become more susceptible to common tennis injuries involving the shoulder, elbow, back, or knee.

Consult with a sports performance specialist to obtain a personalized strength training program that incorporates applicable training technologies for enhanced tennis performance. In addition to building functional strength, a properly designed strength and conditioning training program will also help promote stress relief, facilitate weight management, and improve your overall health.

Participating in a training program that includes these things will help give you a sense of confidence each time you take the court. It's not always going to be easy, but it's definitely going to be worth it. Trust me, the work you put in off the court will pay huge dividends not only on the tennis court, but also on the "court" of your everyday life. Remember, the most successful tennis players are not the ones who hit precise, powerful shots once in a while, but the ones that do it often and consistently throughout the course of a match.

Tennis-specific mental preparedness. As physically demanding as tennis is, it is just as mentally demanding. True success in tennis requires that you have a crystal clear mental picture of the desired outcome and the physical ability to follow through in order to bring it to fruition. Mental training can increase the likelihood of accomplishing your tennis objectives on a more consistent basis. As you are preparing to play, be sure to include mental training, strategy, and visualization techniques to help achieve your peak performance during each match. For more information on mental conditioning, read the following chapters: Champion Steve Cutler, 'The Science of Change – Mental Conditioning;' Champion Tony Books Avilez, 'Mental Conditioning – Self Talk.'

The game of tennis has changed immensely in the past five to ten years. As much as it once was a game of finesse and precision, many players are now almost required to possess tremendous power, blazing speed, amazing athleticism, and laser focus just to be competitive at their respective levels. Just watch women like Venus and Serena Williams, Justine Henin-Hardenne, or men like Andy Roddick, Andre Agassi, and Lleyton Hewitt. While their style of play varies across the board, they all exhibit remarkable strength, exceptional quickness, and extraordinary concentration. These top professional tennis players are taking their play and the game of tennis to the next level; and they're doing it by incorporating tennis-specific strength and conditioning workouts and the right nutritional mix into their training program.

You may not have aspirations to play like the aforementioned pros, but just envision this… You're sitting around before a doubles match showing off your new high-tech racquet to some friends, or comparing outfits with the ladies in your country club's tennis league before taking the court… and everyone is commenting on how nice your racquet is or how cute your outfit looks. But then you get on the court, and your game is horrendous…not because you're a less skillful player, but because your fitness level for tennis leaves much to be desired…oh the embarrassment!

Now imagine the same scenario, only this time when you take the court and begin playing, you're moving effortlessly and hitting precise, powerful shots at will. True Inspiration! Soaring Confidence! Positive Mental Attitude! Shining Example! …and everyone stands in awe because you've taken your game to another level, and you look great doing it! And that's only the beginning…

Robert L. Selders, Jr., CFT, CSCS

214-215-0686
Robert.Selders@thepowerofchampions.com

SECTION EIGHT
Champions Break Barriers!

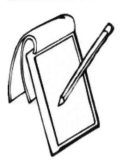

Notes from Phil

The goal is in sight . . . but the path may appear ominous. There may be rocks in the way, boulders that have to be moved, and craters and crevices that must be navigated. Champions see the obstacles, but they see them not as roadblocks. View them as challenges to be recognized, navigated, and overcome.

If the idea of living life as a Champion seems to be a stretch right now, if some of what you've read might apply to "other people," but you're not quite sure it's within the realm of your own capability, summon up what you've already learned about the Mind and Attitude of a Champion. Know that one step at a time can lead you to that goal, and if you have Virus Number "Too," we'll do something about that right now.

Oh, wait a minute, I haven't yet defined the Virus Number "Too." When the "Too" virus infects someone, they begin summoning up words and phrases that manifest as crippling excuses.

"I'm "too" big . . . "

"I'm "too" old . . . "

"I'm "too" out of shape . . ."

While the Attitude of a Champion can quiet the internal voice, you also need specific technologies to defeat the virus fully. You need practical steps to move beyond the next obstacle, and in this section, for those who are "too" something or other, you'll find the tools and strategies to move you away from Virus Number "Too," right up to the finish line . . . . where you can stand as Number "Won."

In addition to the crippling beliefs that can limit the potential for physical improvement, the Champions have also learned to address physical obstacles and challenges that may result from unsupportive lifestyle habits. Champion Katie Mital will begin this section by discussing a common malady that befalls our adult population, the "Ouch, My Aching Back" syndrome. Champion Debi Lander will then share a few ideas that can help individuals who might have been conditioned to believe their physical size might hinder achievement. Then our Champion Doug Carlyle will clear things up for those who might mistakenly believe they're "too old." For those who may perceive that they are just "too busy," Champion Doug Jackson shares some time efficient strategies for making certain your exercise regimen finds its place in your schedule.

My Aching Back by Katie Mital

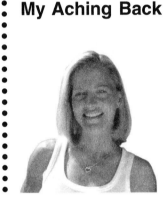

Champion Katie Mital of San Clemente, California specializes in women and adults with special health needs. She has a proven record of successfully creating safe and effective exercise programs to help her clients overcome their personal barriers and achieve a lifestyle of health and wellness.

You're looking forward to getting home after a long, stressful day at work.

As you're leaving your office, you bend over to pick up your briefcase and, when you try to stand up, your lower back spasms, causing you to drop to your knees in pain.

Sound familiar? It is estimated that 80 percent of adults in North America will have at least one episode of back pain sufficiently severe that they lose time from work. The cost of lower back pain in the United States as a result of time lost from work and permanent disability is estimated to be $75 billion per year.[49]

The good news is that most bouts with lower back pain improve quickly. By increasing the strength and flexibility of your "core" region – your lower back, abdominals and legs – you can speed recovery from lower back pain, or even avoid it altogether.

What Causes Lower Back Pain?

The most common causes of lower back pain are strains and sprains. A strain occurs when muscles of the lower back rip or tear. Sprains refer to overstretching of one or more of the ligaments in the back. Lower back strains and sprains are usually due to the application of a heavy load or sudden force to the muscles before they are ready for activity. The Do's and Don'ts defined in Champion Erik Naclerio's chapter, 'Avoiding Injury in the Weight Room,' will help you avoid sprains and strains in the gym. Strains and sprains will normally heal within a short period of time and may never cause further problems.

Another common cause of lower back pain is disc injury. A herniated, or "slipped," disc may bulge out from its position between two vertebrae and may even rupture. A herniated disc compressing a nerve causes sciatica, which is pain that is felt into the buttocks or legs.

Age can also contribute to lower back problems. Wear and tear on your spine causes degeneration in the discs and arthritic changes in the small joints. When these changes are severe, they can cause low back stiffness and pain. Osteoporosis, particularly in post-menopausal women, can contribute to fractured or compressed vertebrae.

There are many causes of lower back pain. If you experience acute pain in your lower back, or you experience pain for more than two to four weeks, see your healthcare practitioner to determine the exact cause and the proper treatment.

Should You Exercise with Lower Back Pain?

There are guidelines you can follow to determine when your lower back pain requires a break in your exercise program:

- If you have seen a healthcare practitioner for back pain in the past, it's a good idea to check with them before you engage in a new exercise program.
- If you have experienced chronic lower back pain for more than two to four weeks, hold off on exercising and make an appointment to see a doctor.
- When you are experiencing acute pain in your lower back, take a break from your workout unless otherwise directed by a healthcare practitioner.
- If you have had back surgery or a recent back injury, follow your physician's plan for rehabilitation before embarking on an exercise program. Following rehabilitation, physicians often recommend an ongoing exercise program. Make sure that your exercise program incorporates recommendations from your physician.
- If it hurts, don't do it! If an activity causes or increases pain in your lower back, skip it.

Follow your physician's recommendations and get back into your fitness routine as soon as possible. An episode of lower back pain should only be a small setback in your exercise program, not an excuse to give it up!

Can Exercise Help You Avoid Lower Back Pain?

Yes. Preventing a back injury is much easier than repairing one. The right exercise and a good stretching program can go a long way in helping you avoid back pain.

Aerobic Exercise

Weight loss is instrumental in relieving pressure on the back and easing or avoiding lower back pain. Aerobic exercise is a key component of weight loss and is often recommended. There are several types of aerobic exercise that are gentle to the back and provide effective conditioning, including walking, stationary bicycling, and water exercise.

Strengthening Exercises

Strengthening the muscles that support the spine will help hold the spine in proper posture and reduce the risk of lower back injury. Weaknesses in the core region are often key contributors to lower back sprains and strains. When these muscles are in poor condition, additional stress is applied to the spine as it supports the body. Strong abdominal and lower back muscles can help speed healing and recovery from lower back pain or injury.

The following exercises will help increase strength in core muscles. Perform each of the exercises two to four times per week after a 5-10 minute warm up. Repeat each exercise ten to fifteen times.

Ab Curl - strengthens abdominal muscles
Lie on back with knees bent, feet flat on floor and hands lightly supporting neck. Squeeze abdominal muscles and slowly raise head and shoulders off the floor until shoulders are about three to five inches off the floor. Hold briefly and lower to starting position.

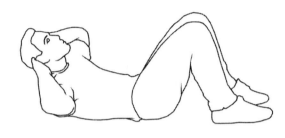

Bridge - strengthens buttocks, leg and back muscles
Lie on back with knees bent and feet flat on floor. Keeping shoulders on floor, squeeze buttocks and lift hips off ground until body forms straight line from shoulders to knees. Hold for three seconds and lower hips back to floor.

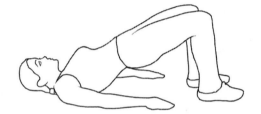

Wall Sit - strengthens back, hip and leg muscles
Stand with stability ball between lower back and wall, or with back directly against wall if stability ball is not available. Feet should be shoulder width apart, heels about 18 inches in front of hips. Slowly bend knees and lower into a "seated" position, keeping back flat. When in the seated position, knees should form a 45 to 90 degree angle and should not go past toes. Hold seated position for a count of five and return to starting position.

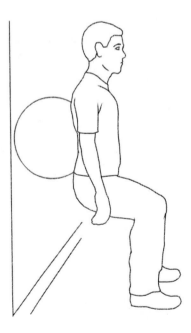

Leg Lifts - strengthens abdominal and hip muscles
Lie on back with arms by sides or resting on your
abs. Keeping lower back flat against floor, lift one
leg off floor and hold for a count of three. Return
leg to floor and repeat movement for other leg.

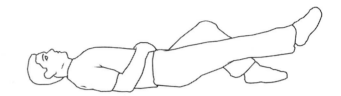

Alternating Arm & Leg Lift - strengthens
abdominal and back muscles
Kneel on hands and knees with knees directly
under hips and palms under shoulders. With
abs tight and without allowing the lower back to
sag, extend left leg back and right arm forward.
Hold briefly and return to kneeling position.
Repeat on the other side.

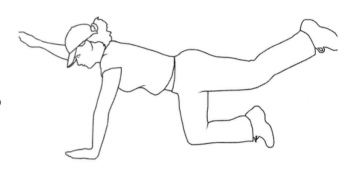

Flexibility Exercises

Stretching the muscles, ligaments and tendons around the spine is crucial to maintaining a strong and healthy
back. The spinal column is designed to move, and tightness can hinder movement, increase stress on the
lower back, and accentuate pain.

Perform the following stretches daily after a 5-10 minute aerobic warm up. Hold each stretch for 20-30
seconds.

Lower Back Stretch
Lie on back with knees bent and feet flat on floor. Place both
hands under knees and gently pull knees as close to chest as
possible.

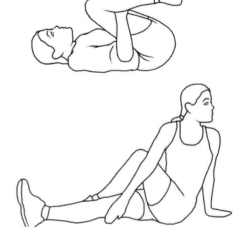

Torso Twist
Sit on floor with legs extended. Cross left leg over right so that
left foot is on outside of right knee. Twist torso to the left,
pressing right elbow against outside of left knee. Repeat on the
other side.

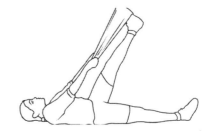

Hamstring Stretch

Lie on floor and loop towel around bottom of one foot. Keeping lower back flat against the floor, raise leg off floor and stretch back of leg. Repeat on other leg.

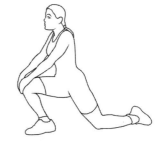

Hip / Groin Stretch

Kneel with right foot in front. Slowly shift weight forward onto right foot and stretch front of left leg. Repeat on other leg.

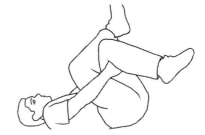

Outer Hip Stretch

Lie on back with bent knees. Cross right leg over left, grasp back of left leg and pull to chest to stretch buttock and hip. Repeat on other leg.

Many adults will experience lower back pain in their lives. While you can't completely eliminate the risk of lower back pain, you can greatly reduce the risk by following a basic strengthening and flexibility program for the core region. Follow these simple suggestions, and you'll enjoy a healthier, more active lifestyle.

Katie Mital, B.S., ACE CPT/CES

Katie Mital Personal Fitness
770 Calle Vallarta
San Clemente, CA 92673
949-369-0929
Katie.Mital@thepowerofchampions.com

Tips for Beginning/Overweight (Obese) Exercisers by Debi Lander

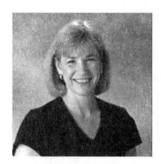

Champion Debi Lander of Jacksonville, Florida is a trainer, public speaker, author and motivational master. She is considered the Pied Piper of Exercise in the Jacksonville area, leading clients to shed unwanted pounds as they follow the path to improved health and fitness.

Congratulations! You've made the big decision to "get fit."

Exercise takes time — you can't do anything to change that! Stop feeling that you don't have the time to spend - your life may depend on this - honestly! Stop feeling guilty that you are taking time away from your family, job or whatever. Just the opposite is true - you are giving those you love a gift by becoming healthy. Don't think of exercise as a perk - it is a necessity for life. Here are some tips to help get you started.

Choosing an Appropriate Exercise

If you are overweight, it adds pressure on your joints so it's best to rule out high impact activities, i.e., running or jumping. Walking is usually the safest and easiest place to start. Where should you walk? Right out your front door may be a good place to start — or not! Is it safe for walking? It's best to find a location with level sidewalks or paths that are away from heavy traffic and fumes. Your local high school track is also a good choice. Malls often allow walkers to use the facility before opening hours. Remember the more convenient your exercise location, the easier it is to stick with it.

Treadmill walking eliminates excuses by providing the opportunity to walk without weather concerns, stray dogs or uneven pavement. It also promotes progressive intensity increases by changing the speed or incline.

Alternatives to walking are cycling and aquatic exercise. Indoor cycling is a great option, assuming you have access to a stationary bike. There are options for turning outdoor bikes into stationary, indoor bikes as well. If you go biking outside, please choose a bike path or other safe location.

Aquatic exercise, lap swimming, water walking, aqua jogging or aqua aerobics classes are easy on the joints but, of course, require a pool and a bathing suit. For some, the bathing suit may be more of an obstacle to overcome than the pool!

Additional and more intense forms of cardiovascular exercise may be added once you have established a consistent program and have no joint problems. This is an important point if weight loss is your goal; you must workout with some intensity to reap the greatest benefits. However, start where you are comfortable and medically safe. If you push too hard, you run the risk of turning yourself off to movement altogether. Forget the quick fix and build your intensity gradually.

Alone, a Partner or Group Workouts?

A lot depends on what you want to accomplish - in addition to burning calories and gaining health benefits. Do you need alone time to think or get away from it all? If so, choose solitary workouts. If you live alone, however, a walking buddy who is supportive and provides motivational force could be helpful. Knowing your buddy is waiting keeps you on track when you don't feel like following your fitness plan. Lastly, a group can provide camaraderie with others who may be at a similar – or higher – fitness level. A weekly schedule that includes solo and group exercise offers the best of both worlds. Variety is a key ingredient to exercise success.

How Long?

It's always best to start small and build from there. Some people may only be able to do 5 -10 minutes the first time out whereas others can do more. Listen to your body. After years of seeing clients experience foot and knee problems, I recommend overweight beginners limit themselves to 30 minutes every other day the first two weeks. It's great when you can't wait to add more exercise but miserable to be suffering with overuse injuries. As your body adapts, add more days (up to 6, with one recovery day) and increase the intensity, pushing you to move faster.

Accountability

Being accountable for your activity is a major factor to success. You need to record and measure your progress. The simplest way is to get a journal and start writing down the date, type of exercise, time it took and the distance covered. Develop a course or neighborhood loop and measure that distance with your car. In a few short weeks you will see that it takes less time to cover the same distance. Don't decrease your exercise time if you finish quicker, keep with about 30 minutes and simply increase your mileage! Additionally ask someone to review your weekly fitness diary. A personal trainer makes a terrific exercise partner!

It's also important to increase daily living activity or non-exercise movement. A pedometer counts your total daily steps or an accelerometer counts your daily movement not just those during exercise. Treadmills and other machines give you feedback data only on workout time.

Strength and Flexibility Training

Exercises to build strength, improve muscle tone and increase flexibility are also necessary for a well-balanced program. Muscle tissue will help burn fat and reshape your body during weight loss. However, starting all these at once may overwhelm and confuse you. Begin by adding stretches at the end of your aerobic workout when your muscles are warm. Ask a fitness professional to demonstrate proper body alignment. Yoga, Pilates and TaiChi classes are future considerations.

After a month of consistent aerobic exercise (or longer if you are still struggling with commitment), begin to add strengthening exercises. The least expensive method is exercise tubing or dumbbells. Have a fitness professional teach you the exercises or use an instructional video at home. Correct form is necessary, so make sure you get it right. Champion Brian J. Johnston's chapter, 'Cultivating Consistency,' can help you stay committed to your exercise program.

Overuse Injuries

If you feel tightness and pain down your lower leg, especially when touched, you may have shin splints. Allow your body time to recover and proceed with care. Pain on the bottom of your feet is another common problem and requires stretching the feet multiple times a day. Wear supportive shoes at all times. Contact a physician if the pain continues.

Transforming from a non-exerciser into a fit and trim person is a long process. Use positive affirmations about getting stronger, mentally and physically each day. Small progressive changes lead to long-term, maintainable goals. See 'Mental Conditioning – Self Talk' by Champion Tony Books Avilez and 'Mental Conditioning – The Science of Change' by Champion Steven Cutler to find out how to effect a positive shift in your thinking.

Additional Tips

Shoes

Do not start your walking program in an old pair of shoes that have been hiding in your closet! Even if you have never used them, the cushioning in sneakers breaks down rather quickly. You need good supportive shoes fitted to your feet. Every step requires your feet, ankles, knees, hips and back to support and absorb the shock from pounding the pavement. Walkers need shoes that have extra shock absorption at the heel as well as soles that provide a good roll off the toes.

Before you go to the store (I recommend an athletic shoe store), you should know if your feet have high, medium, or low arches. To determine, wet the bottom of your bare feet and make footprints on a paper bag. If the forefoot and heel areas are connected by a thin line, you have high-arched feet. If the footprints look pretty much like the shape of your foot, you have a low arch. A medium arch falls somewhere in between.

A high-arched foot is not very flexible so you need a cushioned shoe. If you're flat-footed, your feet are too flexible, and you need a motion control shoe. Those who have medium arches would request something in the middle, often called a stability shoe.

If you have any special foot problems, be sure to mention it to the person fitting your shoes. The American Orthopedic Foot and Ankle Society makes several recommendations:

- Have both feet measured when they are at their largest — at the end of the day or after exercise.
- Wear your workout socks and walk around the store.
- Ensure that the shoe provides at least one thumb's width of space from the longest toe to the end of the toe box.

After 300 to 500 miles, the cushioning on most shoes wears out— sorry but you'll need a new pair! Please take the time and spend the money to get good walking shoes. Part of the struggle of obesity is a poor self-image. Take this step to start building your self-esteem by taking care of your needs.

Sports Bras

All women need to wear a bra during active movement. This is especially true for overweight women. Invest in a sports bra; there are many companies that make them in larger sizes. (Check the Internet or your local sporting goods store.) This might be an expense you hadn't anticipated but, trust me, this is a requirement for success.

If you still feel too bouncy during exercise, I suggest you wear something tight like a leotard, bathing suit or a top with a built in bra over your sports bra. While it may sound a bit strange, it does work. You want to be able to move comfortably with as little bounce as possible.

Chafing

Rubbing or chafing can be a real problem, and you don't want anything to slow you down! Sporting goods stores and running shops carry special lubricants (Body Glide) that don't wear off as quickly as Vaseline or other creams. Apply it to your inner thighs and arms (where the shirt sleeve rubs) and other vulnerable areas before starting your workout. Hopefully your shoes won't give you blisters but, if they do, use a lubricant and band aids in areas needed.

Clothing

One of the surest ways to pick out a beginner in the gym is to look for the person wearing a sweat suit. You can wear that outfit to the gym but you need to be cooler during exercise. Look for special breathable fabrics that wick moisture away from your body. These are much more comfortable than cotton t-shirts. Once again check the Internet for manufacturers of plus size athletic wear, if necessary.

Remember, it took a while for your body to get out of shape - be patient as you work to reshape, tone and improve it. You don't have to jump in all at once. Hang in there and I promise you will get results.

Debi Lander, M.Ed., CSCS, Master Fitness by Phone Coach, ACE LWMC

904-880-2799
Debi.Lander@thepowerofchampions.com
www.healthwisefitness.com

Too Old? by Douglas K. Carlyle

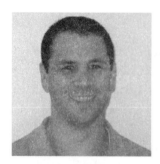

Champion Douglas K. Carlyle of Puyallup, Washington is the owner of Fitness Pros Plus and has been providing fitness training and health education services to athletes, seniors, adolescents and individuals with multiple medical conditions for over 15 years.

A few years ago, I had a conversation with a man that was preparing to run his first marathon (26.2 miles) at the young age of 60.

He had been active in athletics during his high school and college years. After getting out of the Army in his early 20's, he told himself that he would never run for conditioning again. Well, the next decade quickly passed with him staying true to his word. However, while in his thirties, he noticed he had started to gain weight around his midsection. Though jogging around the country roads where he lived was not mainstream, he began to jog a few times a week to combat his expanding waistline. Starting out slowly, he gradually increased to the point where he was jogging regularly, 3-4 miles each day, a few days per week. This exercise regimen continued to be a part of his life for the next 25 years.

By the time he reached his late 50's, he had watched two of his children complete a full marathon. Thinking a marathon may be out of his reach, he set his sights on completing a half-marathon. After properly training, he felt great satisfaction as he crossed the finish line of his first half-marathon. With the successful completion of a few more half-marathon races, he got the desire to take on the challenge of completing a full 26 mile 385 yard marathon.

I will never forget my conversation with this man when he was in the final days of his marathon training. He indicated that he was amazed his body was in condition, at age 60, to do something he could not have physically done at any other time in his life. He realized that if he had trained properly in his 30's, 40's or 50's he could have accomplished a similar feat. However, as a result of sticking to an exercise program, he was now conditioned physically, as a "senior citizen," to run farther than he had ever run at any point in his life!

There are many more stories of older adults accomplishing similar physically demanding feats, not only in their sixties but in their 70's, 80's and even 90's. However, these "seniors" are in the minority. Most seniors accept the decline in strength, balance, flexibility and stamina as an inevitable fate of the aging process. They don't know or believe that "exercise is the closest thing we have to an anti-aging pill."[50] They give little thought to exercise and proper nutrition as important keys to slowing down the decline in physical abilities. They accept their "golden years" as a time to slow down, take it easy, and relax! This new "golden" way of life quickens the aging process! It speeds up the decline in stamina, strength, balance and flexibility. It decreases independence and quality of life.

We Were Made to Move

Have you ever gone on a drive through a small farming community? If you have, I am sure that you have noticed an old car or an old farm truck sitting next to a weather beaten, slightly leaning old barn. Upon seeing these unused vehicles, I have often wondered, "When was the last time that old car moved?" or "Did they expect to park that truck there and never move it again?" A few times I have actually examined some of these old cars and trucks more closely. I have discovered they had much more wear and tear than older models of similar cars and trucks that had been properly used, serviced and maintained. The tires were cracked and oftentimes had gone flat, the paint was faded, many hoses and belts were broken, and the battery was drained and unable to provide the energy necessary to start the car. The lack of service and usage of these old, parked vehicles had speeded up the "aging process." The longer they sat unused, the worse the condition was. However, with a lot of effort and work, restoration of these rundown vehicles is possible.

Your body is a lot like these old, rundown, farm cars and trucks. If you park it and just let it sit, it will deteriorate more quickly than if you properly care for and use it. The longer your body sits without being serviced and used, the worse your conditioning becomes. Your muscles will lose strength and flexibility. Your stability while walking will decrease. The ability of your heart to send blood to the various working parts of your body during simple activities will decrease. Over time, you will lose the ability to perform the basic activities of daily living such as walking, driving, shopping, housework, getting dressed and maintaining proper hygiene. When you lose these abilities, you become dependent on others.

I visited with a lady in her late 70's that had "parked" her body most of the previous decade. She shared an experience with me that illustrated the point, "If we do not use it, we will lose it." She lived by herself in an apartment in an assisted-living facility. One night she got out of bed to use the bathroom. After finishing, she attempted to rise from the toilet and return to bed. However, her legs were too weak for her to stand up. After several unsuccessful attempts at standing up, she had no choice but to remain on the toilet until the cleaning lady arrived the next morning. Embarrassed and sore from sitting on the hard toilet seat for several hours, she wondered if it was time to give up the independence of living alone. She didn't think there was anything that could be done to help her regain some of her lost strength and continue living independently. Fortunately for her, she was wrong! By incorporating a few simple strength training exercises into her life and becoming aware of proper posture while standing, sitting and walking, lost strength was regained. No longer did getting out of a chair or off the toilet require maximum effort.

Too Old?

There is good news!! Research has shown the human body will respond positively to a properly designed exercise program. Even people in their 90's have shown improvements in physical function as a result of regular adherence to an appropriate exercise routine. You can improve your muscle strength, balance which will help prevent falls, coordination and stamina to accomplish not only basic activities of daily living but also recreational activities. Your overall quality of life can be improved dramatically through regular adherence to an appropriately designed exercise program. It is not too late to start exercising and reaping its benefits. The sooner you begin exercising the better chance you have of regaining some of the lost strength, balance and stamina of earlier years. It is possible, with some effort and guidance, to actively enjoy your "golden years."

Douglas K. Carlyle, M.S., CSCS

9609 124th Street East
Puyallup, WA 98373
253-770-5606
Doug.Carlyle@thepowerofchampions.com
www.fitnessprosplus.com

Time Efficient Workouts by Doug Jackson

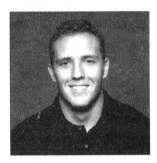

Champion Doug Jackson of Bowling Green, Ohio is the owner of Personal Fitness Advantage, LLC. He writes a free fitness newsletter, 'Fitness Empowerment Monthly,' which you can subscribe to at his website.

Let's face it, we're busy!

In a poll of subscribers to my newsletter, 'Fitness Empowerment Monthly,' ninety percent of respondents stated that lack of time was their biggest obstacle in achieving the fitness results they were looking for. We could get into a debate about whether it's really a time issue or if it's just priorities, but that's another story. My goal is to provide you with both an understanding of how short workouts can fit into a successful fitness lifestyle and share with you the top five strategies you can implement to have an effective and time efficient workout program.

First, it's critically important for people to realize that they can receive many of the benefits of fitness without exercising for hours per day. In fact, many of my clients strength train only twice per week and reap great benefit from those sessions. I'm not trying to say that exercising twice a week is as beneficial as exercising six times per week - it probably isn't. However, the right amount of exercise for each person depends on their goals, genetics, fitness background, external stress level, and other factors.

For many of us, working out more than three or four days per week just doesn't fit into our schedule or match our priorities. In any case, there are diminishing returns with exercise. For example, increasing exercise from three to six times per week will not likely result in a two hundred percent improvement in results. I think that to some extent, the right amount of exercise is the amount of exercise that a person can realistically stick with consistently for a continued amount of time.

With that being said, I do want to be clear about my definition of exercise. When I talk about exercise, I'm not talking about taking a short walk, gardening, walking up some stairs, etc. These physical activities are better than doing nothing at all and will probably help someone maintain a minimal fitness level, but are unlikely to significantly improve their fitness. To find true fitness improvement, scientifically-based exercise sessions that progressively and appropriately become more challenging are necessary so your body continues to adapt.

You must decide on your personal fitness goals and decide how high a priority you will give to these goals. As a minimum, performing two to three exercise sessions per week is necessary to reap the benefits of fitness. Assuming that each session lasts around one hour, this minimum will occupy no more than two percent of the total time in your entire week.

If performing the minimum two or three progressive exercise sessions per week is the maximum time investment you are willing to make at this point, then there are two things that you must be aware of. First, you will not see results as quickly as someone who places fitness as a higher priority and spends more time performing a scientifically-based exercise program. This is okay as long as you realize that this is a lifestyle commitment and reaching fitness goals more slowly is much better than not reaching them at all. Secondly, if you are only working out two or three times per week, you must maximize your time within each of those sessions.

My Top 5 Strategies for Time Efficient Workouts

Workout Planning: First, you need to be clear about your fitness goals. Second, you must have a workout program that is scientifically designed to support the achievement of your goals. After that, you need to mentally prepare for your workout before you begin. Mentally rehearse what you will do during your workout and how you will feel while doing it. Have your workout program designed ahead of time to increase your focus, the effectiveness of your workouts, and save time.

Cut Out the Gym Talk: Those sixty seconds between sets can become five or six minutes if you get caught up in conversations with other gym members. While there's nothing inherently wrong with socializing, if you want measurable results on a time crunch, the small talk must be minimized. When you are focused on the workout, you are less likely to talk to others.

Pick "Big Bang for Your Buck" Exercises: This may be the most important point of all. All exercises are not equal and when time is tight, you want to perform exercises that work a large amount of muscles at the same time. Exercise professionals call these multi-joint exercises. Exercises that don't give you that 'big bang for your buck' are generally single joint exercises. For example, a leg workout that emphasizes multi-joint exercises may take twenty to thirty minutes to perform and will generally be more effective than a lower body workout that emphasizes single joint exercises, which isolate muscle groups, that may take upwards of sixty minutes to complete. When your workouts are on a time crunch, you should emphasize variations of the pushup, squat, deadlift, lunge, chin up or pulldown, row, chest press, and the shoulder press. If you focus on the multi-joint exercises, all muscle groups will be worked in an efficient manner and you will get more exercise progress in less time.

Advanced Training Techniques: If a client of mine is particularly limited in the amount of time they have to train during a given workout, we use particular strategies during the actual workout that drastically decrease the amount of training time. These methods have been used within the bodybuilding world for a long time, but I believe they are just as beneficial for general fitness when you are trying to perform an effective workout with limited time. These methods include supersets, descending sets, and forced repetitions. Please note that these methods place a lot of strain on the body and should not be used every day.

During a superset, you will go from one exercise to another with little or no rest. We use this strategy when working two opposing muscle groups during the same workout. For example, if you are training the chest and upper back, you may alternate between chest presses and rows.

Descending sets take the exhaustion of a muscle to a further level. During this strategy, you may combine three or four sets of the same exercise in a row. For example, instead of taking 10 minutes to complete three sets of ten repetitions on a row with rest periods in between, you would start with a normal first set. When completed with that set, immediately and with no rest, decrease the amount of weight used on the exercise and continue with another 5-8 repetitions. Normally you would repeat this same procedure for a third time as well.

Forced reps are another technique that further exhaust the muscle in a quick manner. Simply have someone help you with 1-2 more repetitions that you complete after reaching momentary muscle failure.

All of these advanced techniques help you train the muscle in a time efficient manner while still stimulating muscular adaptation so you continue to see fitness improvement.

Try Interval Training: Interval training is an effective and high-intensity form of cardiovascular conditioning that does not take as long as traditional cardiovascular training programs. Simply put, when you interval train, you alternate between high and low intensity during cardiovascular exercise. The combination of the physiological effects from the high intensity parts of the workout along with the benefits of increased duration provided by the lower intensity parts of the workout allow you to get the best of both worlds. This is the way to get a 'big bang for your buck' with cardiovascular training.

There's different ways to perform the intervals. I simply like to alternate between higher and lower intensity running every thirty seconds (a 1:1 ratio between high/low intensity work). Other fitness pros will discuss working at 1:2 or 1:3 ratios. Find what works for you. I'd suggest starting out at only 10-12 minutes of work (5-6 minutes high intensity and 5-6 minutes at a lower intensity while alternating every 30 seconds) and increasing one minute per week until you reach 30-40 minutes. If you are on a time crunch, simply perform 10-15 minutes of interval training at the end of your strength training session.

With the appropriate application and integration of these behavioral and exercise science strategies, you should be able to increase your exercise effectiveness while decreasing your time in the gym. Just remember that you don't have to spend hours upon hours in the gym to find fitness achievement and its corresponding rewards to other areas of your life.

Doug Jackson, CSCS, ACE

Personal Fitness Advantage
Bowling Green, Ohio
419-260-9064
Doug.Jackson@thepowerofchampions.com
www.personalfitnessadvantage.com

SECTION NINE
Champion "Down Time"

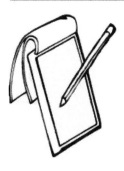

Notes from Phil

Stress is a word we're all familiar with, and we usually think of stress as being detrimental. It can be; however, exercise is stress and, if the body is allowed to go through beneficial cycles of stress periods and recovery periods, that stress becomes a stimulus toward positive change. When our bodies are under stress, the adrenal glands increase production of a hormone called cortisol. This hormone allows our body to break down tissue so that tissue can be rebuilt with new healthy cells. When cortisol levels are elevated continuously, without the recovery period allowing for other hormones to positively impact protein synthesis, fat release, and brain function, our bodies begin a gradual process of deterioration. It's vital that we get adequate exercise, but it's every bit as important that we allow our bodies to relax and recuperate.

I know what you're thinking. We're busy. We have jobs. We have families. We have obligations. Relaxation is a luxury we can't afford. I think journalist Sydney J. Harris made a very good point when he stated, "The time to relax is when you don't have time for it." Relaxation and downtime are not as much luxuries as they are needs. This book is intended to empower you as well as to help you readjust your mindset, and now it's time to better understand the healing art of relaxation.

In this section, Champion Sandy Rusch will help you identify the signs of overtraining. She'll then provide you with strategies to make certain you keep the stress-recovery cycles in balance. Champion Jason Brice follows on the theme of recovery by pointing out some common mistakes and sharing some real-world measures for optimizing recovery.

Overtraining: Too Much of a Good Thing by Sandy Rusch

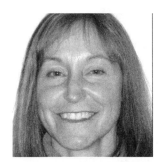

Champion Sandy Rusch of Madison, Wisconsin is a 25 year fitness professional veteran. She founded Fitness Balance in 1995, the premiere Personal Training, Pilates Studio in Madison with an emphasis on fitness and wellness for women.

Americans are being bombarded with the message that we are overweight as a result of inactivity.

The statistics are compelling. More than sixty percent of us are now overweight or obese, which experts are calling an epidemic.

There are two sides to every coin, however, and just as inactivity creates health problems, too much exercise carries its own dangers. The athlete who works out 2-3+ hours seven days a week may be setting themselves up for overtraining or the "staleness syndrome." A syndrome is a cluster of symptoms, behaviors and conditions that can lead to disease or, in the case of overtraining, "dis-ease." For example, you have been committed to your cardio, strength and flexibility programs spending 2 hours running, 90 minutes with weights and another hour in Pilates or yoga class. You feel like you should be fitter than ever. Instead your hamstrings are always sore, your runs are slower and you can't improve that bench press. This type of training stress can lead to overtraining. It is directly correlated to exercise addiction but the purpose of this chapter will address overtraining as it relates to volume of exercise and the problems it can create.

In 1975, a seasoned running coach told me, "Always train for a marathon…but never actually run one." He believed that the physical and mental rigors of completing a 26.2 mile race set one up for overtraining, overextending and exhaustion. Marathon training programs have changed and improved since then but it was food for thought then and now.

Some 54 years ago, Roger Bannister broke the 4 minute mile mark, arguably one of the finest physical achievements of mankind. He accomplished this by training 30 minutes a day! Obviously he was an athlete with great talent, genetics and a training program that worked well for him. Many believed this was the peak or pinnacle of effort and a record not to be broken. However, in the last 10 years, many human performance records have been broken by both men and women. Some contributing factors for this include:

- sports technology
- equipment
- injury rehab
- nutrition
- coaching improvements

Remember 1972 when Mark Spitz won 7 gold Olympic medals? His training consisted of 10,000 yards/5 miles a day, an unheard of volume at that time. Nowadays it is standard for 12 and 13 year olds to do this exact same volume in swimming programs across the US!

Unfortunately, with this increase in volume of exercise and with sports like marathon running and triathlons growing in participation by almost 50%, it is becoming apparent the pathology and physiology of overtraining are not well understood. Indicators of overtraining like mood changes and frustration are difficult to measure and can't be monitored by blood or urine tests. In fact, at this time physicians have no exact criteria for diagnosing overtraining. Dr. Erik Adams, a University of Wisconsin Sports Medicine Physician in Madison, WI, says that patient training logs and ruling out other illnesses is the best method for diagnosing overtraining. Adams says, "ACSM talked about diagnostic blood tests a few years ago but that hasn't caught on and one's mood and performance change are the best indicators."

If you are a highly trained athlete spending many hours a week exercising, prevention of overtraining should be carefully considered. Manipulating and periodizing a training program to vary volume, frequency, intensity and even the kind of exercise performed is essential. Heavy training, even if it is team training, must be looked at individually. Also, recovery days are just as important as active days and must be thoughtfully included in everyone's training program.

Overtraining, when defined loosely, can happen to anyone who achieves an imbalance between activity and recovery in their training lifestyle. However, beginning athletes are typically sidelined more often by overuse or biomechanical injuries vs. the metabolic/psychological issues in overtraining. The overtraining syndrome is more applicable to highly conditioned individuals. If one is practicing a high volume of exercise and maintaining it for an extended period of time, symptoms of overtraining staleness may set in. Signs of overtraining include:

- decreased and impaired physical performance
- possible change in resting heart rate and blood lactate levels (but is not highly predictable)
- frustration and lack of desire for training
- increased musculoskeletal injuries
- increased colds, infections and immune system impairment
- lack of appetite (after eating many calories each day to maintain exercise)
- unusual weight loss
- irritability, anxiety, depressive moods, frustration
- insomnia or changed sleep patterns

If an athlete experiences three or more of these, it is probably time to evaluate the ratio of training time vs. recovery time. Covert Bailey in his book, *Smart Exercise*, describes a study looking at nine ultra-long-distance runners who participated in a ten day, seventeen-mile-a-day race. Each runner had their thighs measured before and after the race. By the end of the race quadriceps size decreased in every runner. It is believed that with little or no recovery time for the muscles to repair and rebuild, the muscles broke down. They weren't capable of rejuvenating. The runners needed some days off! An important fact to emphasize about training is that muscles repair and strengthen after the hard work is done. Training is the set up for the strengthening process. Recovery plays a critical role in human performance improvement.

Moderation and balance in life and training, more often than not, are the best paths to take to prevent overtraining. A client of mine was obsessed with training her triceps to avoid dreaded "teacher arms." She trained them everyday, against my wishes and tried heavy weight and various exercises. No change. Finally she agreed that she was overtraining them. She cut back her triceps work and quickly developed the tone she was missing. Less, if done intelligently, really can be more when it comes to training.

What should an athlete do if he/she experiences a dramatic mental or physical collapse, staleness or displays other overtraining symptoms? The best thing is to step back from the high intensity program for a minimum of 2 weeks. Be aware that overtraining can require up to a year of recovery time. Chris Carmichael, Lance Armstrong's coach, suggests a six week recovery program that takes cardio and strength work down several notches. He recommends 20-30 minutes of easy cardio 2-3 times a week with sit ups, pushups and stretching in small doses performed other days of the week.

Mood is the best determinate of when training should begin again or increase. Any increase should be done slowly. The angst an athlete might feel by stopping exercise altogether could be almost as serious as overtraining. Carmichael's recommended 6 weeks might be helpful. But preventing overtraining should be strived for and practiced diligently.

Training schedule and adequate recovery go hand in hand. Objective indicators for diagnosing overtraining are difficult to prove. One's heart rate may go up or down as could blood lactate levels. Mood and frustration of the athlete tell the tale. Most coaches working with highly trained athletes strive for maximum volume and intensity intended to result in outstanding performance. Recovery time must be included in the equation. Coaches should be always tuning in to their athletes and asking them how they feel. If an athlete is self-coaching, preventing overtraining can be done by self-monitoring and watching mood swings, sleep, diet and tracking all of this in a training log including taper days, rest days after hard days, periodizing so that periods of weeks are spent in a recovery fashion.

The critical factor in overtraining, as in life, is finding the balance. "The same is true of running and wrestling. Thus a master of an art avoids excess and defect (overuse): but seeks the intermediate and chooses this – the intermediate not in the object but relative to us." Aristotle

Be the master of what you do but not to the high or low of losing balance. Remember the best word in fitness is balance.

Sandy Rusch, M.A., ACE

Fitness Balance, Inc.
7606 Westward Way
Madison, WI 53719
608-827-5410
Sandy.Rusch@thepowerofchampions.com

Rest and Recovery from Exercise by Jason Brice

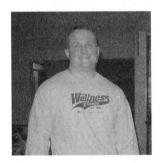

Champion Jason Brice of Rogersville, Tennessee holds a bachelor's degree in Community Health Education from the University of Tennessee. He has won two world drug-free powerlifting championships and is a former high school football All-American. Jason has seven years' experience personal training.

One of the most important aspects of a healthy lifestyle is proper rest and recovery from exercise.

Your gains in fitness come while you are resting, not when you are exercising. Without taking proper steps to recover from exercise, all your hard work may be in vain. You must make sure that you are allowing yourself to fully recover between exercise sessions or you will quickly start to overtrain or injure yourself.

The most important means of recovering from exercise is proper sleeping habits and supportive nutrition. Mistakes in one of these two factors will rob you of the benefits you are working hard for when you exercise. Other methods of speeding up recovery that are often used, and unfortunately often misused or misunderstood, are massage, whirlpools, and saunas.

Sleep

Sleep, especially stage four deep sleep, is when the body best recovers from exercise and is of vital importance. You should get 7-8 hours of sleep each night. If anything in your life is preventing this, eliminate it! Television is probably the worst culprit when it comes to lack of sleep. If there are any television programs that keep you up at night, you need to learn to use a VCR or Tivo and record them to watch later. Do not let anyone (other than a newborn) or anything rob you of your sleep. Lack of sleep will interfere with every single aspect of your life. If your job demands that you regularly sacrifice a good night's sleep, it is simply asking for too much. You will never be as healthy as you should be unless you are getting enough sleep. Even partial sleep deprivation reduces immunity and will prevent you from benefiting as much from exercise as you normally would.

There are a few common mistakes made when it comes to sleeping. One is the use of caffeine. I sometimes hear clients say that they can "drink caffeine just before bedtime and sleep like a baby." It is still unwise to drink caffeine within a few hours of going to bed even if it does not disturb your sleep. Caffeine does not kick in until long after being digested and this will disrupt the precious stage four sleep, rendering it shallow and ineffective.[51] Eating a high carbohydrate meal just before bedtime will disturb sleep as well. A hot bath just before bedtime can induce sleep faster and increases deep sleep. The bedroom should be cool, dark, and quiet.

Showering

A shower should be taken after every workout. Research has shown that alternating 1 minute of hot water (99-100°F) followed by 5-10 seconds of cool water (54-59°F) speeds up recovery more than a shower of constant temperature.[51] Rubbing the worked muscles while in the shower also helps. Ending a shower with cool water is invigorating and useful if taken in the morning or when you have other activities planned after working out. A long, hot shower will help to relieve muscle tension, leaves a feeling of relaxation and is great just before going to sleep.

Nutrition

In order to get optimal results from your workouts, you must eat correctly. You should always eat a supportive meal within 45 minutes after a workout. This drives glycogen and amino acids that were depleted during the workout into the muscles. Eating a junk food diet will not produce the results that supportive eating will. If you are working out, then you have done the hard part. Why throw it away by bad eating habits?

Outdoors

Getting outdoors at least 30-60 minutes every day is also a good idea. Sunshine lowers blood pressure, soothes pain, and stimulates metabolism. Getting outside on cloudy days improves lung ventilation and improves the cardiovascular system. These influences are even more intensive at lower temperatures.[51] Getting outdoors and enjoying nature is also great for relieving stress and has great psychological benefits.

So far I have discussed things that can be done year round in your efforts to fully recover and benefit from your exercise sessions. Now I will discuss a few other ways of enhancing recovery. Unlike what I have discussed so far, the following techniques should not be used all the time. For example, one of the most common mistakes people make using whirlpools is that they use them year round. The body adapts to any means of recovery just like it adapts to using the same exercise program all the time. When the body adapts to a means of recovery, the means used will be rendered ineffective for speeding up recovery. This is why you should change your recovery plan just like you change your workout program from time to time.

I wouldn't recommend most of the following means of recovery for beginners. You want your body to become proficient at recovering from workouts on its own before you start introducing ways of speeding up recovery. I would recommend using the most intensive ways of speeding up recovery during the most intensive phases of training.

Whirlpool/Sauna

Whirlpools and saunas are commonly used to try to enhance workout recovery. Unfortunately, they are commonly misused. Studies done on athletes have shown that using a whirlpool or sauna right after workout (within 3 hours) will speed up recovery above normal the evening it is used but by the next day the recovery rate was actually below the rate of not using a sauna at all. If the whirlpool or sauna was used nine hours after the workout, however, the next day recovery rate was above normal.[52] (Normal here refers to having not used any means of trying to speed up recovery.)

Massage

Massage is another common way of speeding up recovery. Different types of massage have different effects on the body. On the most basic level, massage will help to remove lactic acid and by-products produced by the body while exercising as well as help to bring oxygen and nutrients to the muscle cells to aid recovery. Massage is best done in between workout days, with 24 hours before the next workout. Drinking water after massage helps to rid the body of lactic acid and toxins also.

High Rep Sets (end of exercise)

Ending a heavy workout with a set of high reps and light weights helps saturate the area with blood and helps eliminate some (but not all) of next day muscle soreness. I usually recommend using about 30-40% 1 repetition max (RM).

Conclusion

In order to get optimal benefit from exercise, you must take steps to recover from exercise properly. Good sleep and nutritional habits should be used year round. Other ways to speed up recovery can be used if done correctly and not used too often.

Jason Brice, B.S., CSCS

1183 Stanley Valley Rd
Rogersville, TN 37857
423-431-6668
Jason.Brice@thepowerofchampions.com

SECTION TEN
The "She" Champion

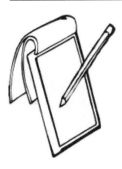

Notes from Phil

For those of you who are old enough (as I am), you remember Billy Jean King defeating "a man" to cement her undisputed place as a Champion. Since then the list of undisputed female champions is virtually endless, and it continues to grow by the day. You no doubt recognize the names, Dominique Moceanu (gymnastics champion), Mia Hamm (soccer champion), Jackie Joyner-Kersee (track and field champion), and Michelle Kwan (figure skating champion). Equality in physical prowess and achievement between the sexes is more a reality than ever in history, and many previously male-dominated sports have opened their doors for "women's leagues," ensuring that new female Champions will emerge. Of course, as our female readers begin to achieve their own goals, they will proudly enter the category of female Champions . . . but despite the open door for equality in performance, there are some differences in male and female biochemistry that might add an element of frustration to our aspiring female Champions.

I'm treading on dangerous ground here, as I'm nearing no-man's land . . . . the mythological place where men "really" understand women. Rather than trusting that I fully understand the female psyche, I've asked some of our Champions, who have the estrogen / testosterone balance swaying in the female direction, to help our female Champions achieve their absolute best. (Oh, and guys, you can read this section too. Everything we learn about women helps. We'll never get to complete understanding, but let's at least give it our best shot!)

Before Champion Kelli Calabrese reveals some fat burning secrets specific to women, Champion Tracy Bloom will blow away the flawed belief that suggests women are somehow "stuck" after 40.

With Champion Karen Webster then taking the reins, we'll go on to understand what women are really looking for when they say, "I don't want to get big, I just want to get toned."

Next Champion Angela Ursprung will reveal why she's earned the nickname, "The Body Sculptress," as she shares some specialization routines focused on the issues that most plague women. Angela then hands the baton to Champion Darrell Morris so he can prove that even male fitness professionals can be adept at teaching women to shape their hips and thighs.

The Student Was Ready . . . At 40! by Tracy Bloom

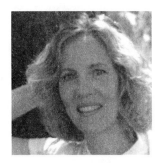

Champion Tracy T. Bloom of Weston, Connecticut has learned firsthand how to make healthy lifestyle changes to achieve her goals. Once weighing more than 200 pounds, she is now a Licensed Massage Therapist and participates regularly in triathlons. A mother of three young children, Tracy trains clients at the local YMCA and in her home studio.

In 1998, at age forty, I lost 60 lbs. and have kept it off for 6 years.

I did it with diet and exercise - no magic bullet. It took about 9 months, at about 1-2 lbs. per week, which is considered to be a healthy rate of weight loss. I did it with the help of my personal trainer. Let me share my story with you.

My neighbor Susan and I have lived in the same small town for years. We had our respective three children each at about the same time and we had both put on a lot of "mommy" weight. As I was dropping my eldest off at school one morning, I noticed a woman stepping lightly up the stairs into the building, her yellow raincoat and long brown hair billowing behind her like flags. She was going up those stairs faster than most people go down.

It was Susan, and she looked incredible! I sat there thinking had that been me climbing those few steps (at 200+ lbs.) I would have been struggling, gasping, and secretly wishing for a towrope like they had on the bunny hill at Butternut before I reached the top! When she came out, I got out of my car and shuffled over to hers. Dripping in the rain, I knocked on her car window. She rolled it down. "Susan, you look fantastic!" I blurted out, "I don't know what you're doing but I want to do it too!"

She said she was working out with a personal fitness trainer and seeing a nutritionist. I demanded their names and phone numbers on the spot and waited in the rain as she found a scrap of paper and wrote down the information. I had made up my mind to change. It happened in a flash.

There is a saying; 'When the student is ready, the teacher appears.'

Over the next few years I learned what it was like to exercise like I never had before. Getting up at 5:00 a.m. for three grueling workouts a week at 5:45 and walking for 20-30 minutes three times a week. All that sweat and you can bet I wasn't going to mess it up by eating junk. I was working too hard and paying too much, and besides, I had made a decision that it was time to get back to my old self.

Call it a mid-life crisis, but I was hell-bent for fitness! My personal trainer, Phil H., had a small private gym in the basement of a small house. He was a powerlifter with several national and state records, so he trained lifting. It was so important to have the support of my trainer! Together, we set goals for my program and achieved them. As a result, at age forty one, I entered and qualified for my first powerlifting meet. I started playing tennis again and had a rocket serve. Recently I completed three triathlons. It was fun being fit!

It was so helpful and necessary to have someone else care whether or not I lost one pound, one inch, or made it through another set of 100 squat thrusts. My success was his success, and when he said I was "pretty hard core," I beamed. He would introduce me as someone who had worked hard and succeeded.

I decided to go to massage school. Learning about the human body was fascinating, so while in school, I got my ACE certification as a personal trainer and continued to study fitness. I wanted to help others as Phil had helped me - I wanted them to experience success!

Now I am a licensed massage therapist and have developed my own way of training, gleaned from everything I've ever studied. I have also started a weight loss and fitness program called WalkBuddy to help support the goals of others who want to get in shape. I train clients both privately and at the local YMCA.

Change isn't always easy. If being fit were easy, then everyone would be in shape. An extremely significant determining factor for creating success is - the turning point. There is a moment when the decision to change occurs. This is often a moment of clarity, a moment of truth, when they fully accept what they need to do.

From then on, these people are unstoppable. This doesn't mean they don't have setbacks and plateaus. There is a commitment to fitness and health as a way of life. They set goals and don't stop until they reach them.

A crucial factor is support - having those around you who recognize your successes and help you reach your goals. It helps to have a trainer who has actually met their own fitness challenges.

Another key factor in my success was changing my relationship with food. I wasn't "on a d**t." I became committed to giving myself the good stuff. I no longer finished my kids' leftover PB & Js. I made myself a healthy lunch. I looked for healthy choices.

I took the time and spent the money to have a salad with chicken instead of pizza. I carried hard-boiled eggs and cottage cheese in a cooler. I was eating often but eating well and never skipped breakfast, which was my biggest meal of the day. Boy, I sure did look forward to those big steaming bowls of hot cereal and fruit and several eggs!

My husband and I used to have a little ritual - a bowl of ice cream every night at 11:00 while watching Seinfeld and laughing until we cried! When I began getting up very early to go to the gym, this late rendezvous with Haagen-Dazs was no longer an option. We started going to bed earlier and, coincidentally, found new little rituals to enjoy together!

Instead of struggling with food, it became a tool to grow my new healthy body. Generally, when I was hungry, I ate. But I trained myself, like I was training my body, to make healthy choices. Life is all about choices. Each time I ate, I was making a choice. And I knew what the consequences would be for continuing habitually wrong choices!

There was no scale at my house, but there was at the gym, and every week I would weigh myself (with Phil looking on) to find out if I had progressed. Success felt wonderful! Once in a while I would plateau, or actually gain a pound, and Phil and I would discuss how to tighten up the program.

While the motivation was mine, as was the commitment, my personal trainer matched my drive and determination with his experience and knowledge - the tried and true - to help me achieve results without wasting my time, money, and resolve.

I am proud to be a member of this group of Champions. Many people have been inspired by my story. It is powerful because it is true. Health can be achieved, and with it comes vitality and an appreciation for life. So take that step; accept your challenge and don't ever stop. Walk your walk.

"Knowledge….the wing wherewith we fly to heaven." Shakespeare

Tracy T. Bloom, ACE, LMT

Weston Massage and Fitness Center
203-226-1797
Tracy.Bloom@thepowerofchampions.com

Fat Burning Secrets for Women by Kelli Calabrese

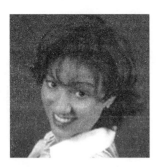

Champion Kelli Calabrese of Long Valley, New Jersey has been successfully helping clients reach their physical goals through a multi-disciplinary approach for almost 2 decades. She is the co-author of *Feminine, Firm & Fit - Building a Lean, Powerful Body*.

It's not in your mind, ladies - men and women do not live in an equal world when it comes to body fat.

Men, with their taller bodies, larger muscles and bones, lay claim to a faster metabolism. At puberty, girls put on fat and boys put on muscle. From fertilization to breastfeeding, women have and need more fat than men. As you read on, keep in mind that, although the odds may appear to be stacked against us, you can overcome stubborn fat and make improvements to your shape and health. First, a brief explanation of the fat burning challenges women face, and then the secrets to overcoming them.

Body Fat Distribution

Women bear almost double the amount of body fat as men, primarily to help them carry and nourish babies. Fat is the major energy source needed for fetal development and protection and we have no control over where the fat cells decide to swell and shrink.

The fat cells in the lower body, where women tend to put on inches, are more prone to fat storage. The fat cells in the upper body, where men tend to carry extra weight, are more prone to releasing fat. Women who have dieted will notice as they lose weight that body fat starts melting away from the upper body first, followed by the persevering lower body fat.

Yet the reverse is true when gaining weight. The fat cells in the hips, thighs, butt and abs will enlarge first. If you see a woman who has yo-yo dieted for years, you will notice her upper body is disproportionately smaller than her lower body.

Hormones

During pregnancy and the menstrual cycle, hormones encourage water retention in the fat cells. The excess fluid slows down circulation and makes it even more difficult to mobilize fat.

The hormone progesterone, which is higher in women than in men, affects appetite and mood. It makes you hungrier during the second half of your menstrual cycle and is responsible for the ravenous appetite you may experience during pregnancy. Progesterone can also make you feel sluggish, sleepy and therefore less inclined to exercise. Women who take birth control pills gain on average 3-5 pounds as a side effect.

Pregnancy

Throughout pregnancy, fat cells in a woman's body not only expand, but often multiply in number. When the pregnancy is over, those fat cells remain and are always ready to enlarge when the body takes in more calories than it uses. In addition, the thyroid gland, which drives the metabolism, becomes notoriously sluggish during pregnancy to help the body hold onto fat. Not surprisingly, after two or three children, the weight loss dilemma may be compounded.

Menopause

During peri-menopause (the 10 years prior to menopause), women begin producing less estrogen, which is a protective hormone. We also begin to sleep less while our appetite becomes stimulated. As peri-menopause begins, fat tends to accumulate around the waist and chest, increasing our risk of heart disease.

Aging

Beginning in the mid-20's, women lose an average of 5 pounds of muscle mass each decade until menopause when it accelerates to 7 pounds per decade.[53] Additionally, non-exercising women typically gain 1-2 pounds of fat a year - for life. And the fat gain can be much higher depending on lifestyle choices.

So, by your mid-40's, you could have lost up to 15 pounds of metabolically active muscle and replaced it with over 20 pounds of sluggish fat – and that's conservative! Your metabolism has dramatically slowed and your body composition has changed in unfavorable proportions.

To make matter worse, if you have tried to diet (I imagine you've attempted one or two), you have likely accelerated the muscle loss process. Dieting without exercise can lead to a 25-28% muscle loss.[54]

Aging also makes excess fat harder to hide. As skin begins to lose its elasticity and sag, it has a harder time containing fat cells, giving the skin a rippled appearance often referred to as cellulite.

Why Men Have It Easier

Testosterone stimulates bone and muscle growth. Men don't lose testosterone as fast as we lose estrogen. Men have more muscle, more bone minerals, and tend to eat about 35% more calories than women. Men also respond faster to exercise training.

Although men don't generally live as long as women, they start and end with more bone, more muscle and more testosterone than women. By the time a woman is 60 years old, she probably has 20 to 30 pounds of muscle on her frame – if she's not exercising.

Women also face many social and emotional challenges, which can lead them to become a slave to the scale, avoid exercise for fear of bulking up and fall for spot reduction and quick fix solutions, all of which only compound the problem. These fears, misconceptions and bugaboos, which hold so many women hostage, could easily fill a book, but let's talk about solutions that do work.

Now that you understand the special physiological challenges women face, here's how to overcome them so you can have the strong, trim, fit body you really want.

Exercise is the key to fat burning. If you do one thing, incorporate 2-3 strength training and 3-5 cardio workouts into your weekly routine using my top 10 fat-burning secrets for women. The results are guaranteed!

- Warm up before a strength training session – I'll bet you never thought this would make a difference, but it really will help you get more out of your workout. Warming up increases blood flow to muscles by about 55% giving you better muscle contraction. You will sweat earlier, which helps to regulate your body temperature. Your warm up will also jump start the neuromuscular connection, which initiates the release of carbohydrate, fat enzymes and hormones while reducing your perceived exertion during strength training. Just 5 minutes of walking or cycling will meet this requirement.

- Vary your cardio exercises – Alternate between two or more cardiovascular activities, such as walking, cycling, kickboxing and step aerobics. This will help to optimally develop your cardiovascular fitness, maintain the element of fun in exercise and help you avoid repetitive injuries. Bottom line - you will expend more calories.

- Incorporate several cardio techniques – Use a combination of continuous, interval, circuit and speed play training. Changing techniques forces your body to adapt and become more efficient. Vary the intensity and modify impact styles. For example, if you have been walking the same path at the same pace every day, begin to incorporate bursts of acceleration intermittently. The underlying principle is that change is what keeps the body progressing, making improvements and burning fat.

- Plan your workouts in phases – Organize your workouts into a cyclic structure. For example, for two to three weeks, exercise at a lower intensity for 45 to 60 minutes, and then, for the next two to three weeks, engage in 20 to 30 minutes at your highest intensity. The following 2 to 3 weeks go at a moderate intensity for 30 to 45 minutes. You can also try a transition week where you perform light amounts of exercise 2 to 3 times weekly for 20 to 25 minutes. This system allows you to maintain a high level of fitness and not overtrain. This cycling of workout structures will help your body become more efficient at fat burning. Champion Brian Schiff describes this type of workout, called periodization, in greater detail.

- Circuit train – Perform several strengthening exercises interspersed with short cardio segments. For example, perform a leg press, lateral pull down and abdominal crunch followed by 3 minutes of cycling. Then repeat another 3 strength exercises followed by 3 minutes of walking. Circuit training has a lower dropout rate, is an efficient calorie burner, increases muscular strength and decreases body fat.

- Strength train with multi-joint exercises – Choose exercises that work compound muscle groups – meaning more than one muscle group at a time. This will give you the most mileage per exercise. Examples include squats, lunges, and pushups. Strength training is what builds muscle and ultimately drives your metabolism. For every pound of muscle on your body you need 35 to 50 calories per day to sustain it, while every pound of fat on your body requires only a modest 2 calories per day.[55]

- Exercise first thing in the morning – Morning exercisers have a higher likelihood of sticking to their program. Later in the day, the odds that you'll skip your workout increase as interruptions arise and fatigue sets in. Morning exercise also helps regulate your hormone response, telling your body to release fat and kick start your metabolism.

- Eat a "primer" meal prior to working out – Having a small balanced meal prior to exercise will help you have the energy to give your workout your best effort and workout more intensely. After you eat, your blood sugar rises and exercise acts like insulin to help regulate blood glucose. Choose to eat balanced whole foods one hour prior to your workout.

- Eat 5 to 6 small meals a day – Food has a thermic effect, meaning it takes energy (calories) for your body to digest the food you eat. Eating several times throughout the day increases the thermic effect so you burn more calories. Eating more often also keeps you from feeling like you are being deprived of food and prevents hunger from setting in. As you may know, going too long without food causes you to binge eat. In short, the grazing approach to eating helps to maximize your fat burning potential throughout the day. My fellow Champions further explain the benefits of eating more frequently in Section 6, 'Eat Like a Champion.'

- Train with intensity – To get the full benefits of exercise, you must graduate from the "pink weights" and moderate walking. Don't be afraid to increase your resistance and challenge your muscles and cardiovascular system. In order to change, you have to push beyond the physical limits you are accustomed to.

You really can attain a feminine, firm, fit and younger appearance regardless of your age or inherited traits. You can overcome any weaknesses and trouble spots to a certain degree with balanced and symmetrical strength, cardiovascular and flexibility training, combined with making nutritious food choices.

Focus on being the best you can be. A lean and healthy body is both realistic and achievable.

Kelli Calabrese, MS, CSCS, ACE

Calabrese Consulting, LLC
908-879-1469
Kelli.Calabrese@thepowerofchampions.com
www.KelliCalabrese.com

Toning by Karen Webster

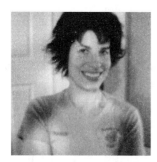

Champion Karen Webster of Furlong, Pennsylvania, trainer, educator, is the co-owner of The Body Works Studio located in the heart of Bucks County, Pennsylvania. Her ultimate mission is to educate and empower women to transform their bodies in a compassionate manner.

Women often think about losing excess weight...and *then* getting toned.

I remember thinking along similar lines as well for many years. Before I became a fitness professional in 1997, I was a 'seasoned' exerciser for 17 years. At that time, I was *thirsty* for knowledge; I read every book I could get my hands on that pertained to diet and exercise and applied what I read. However, all my "efforts" left me with a nagging feeling that it was way too much work for such little payback. What I didn't know was that my luck was about to change!

Enter Synergy

Then it happened. Phil Kaplan was a guest on a local radio station that I normally tuned in to during my early morning commute. As I said, I was not a newcomer to exercise; quite the contrary! I tried step aerobics, workout videos, long-distance power walks, running, and even strength training. I didn't have a weight problem, but I still wasn't pleased with the shape of my thighs; I felt both uncomfortable, and even a bit bottom heavy. Despite my exercising efforts, my legs were flabby.

...Getting back to Phil Kaplan. He delivered his message on the principles of Synergy with such amazing insight and clarity that I finally understood for the first time *why* I wasn't getting the results I was seeking, after all these years. *Aha!* I finally understood why my legs were lacking any real muscle tone. My exercising efforts had completely missed many of the vital components that were necessary to transform my body. Simply put — I was missing the Synergy!

Seeing Both Sides

As both a fitness professional and one-time consumer, I'd like to share some of the insights I've discovered along the way that have helped me achieve my goals. The advice I'm going to share deals with one's mental state. *Open* your mind to being educated if your desire is *permanent* fat loss. Forget what you think you already know about weight loss and instead get ready to embrace what Phil Kaplan refers to as "the fitness truth." Within this truth, ladies, lies the secret to getting that "toned" body we are all striving for! When new clients enter our studio for their first visit, they are usually astounded once they understand the simplicity of this approach. Once you learn to "take control," and apply these principles consistently, you will start to understand that you really *are* in charge of your metabolism.

Toning 101

First, I'd like you to think about the word '*toned*.' What does 'getting toned' really mean? I remember what I thought it meant at one time. Toned meant sort of rearranging or pushing the fat around into a more appealing shape, and of course, losing some of the excess! I hope you find some humor in my response. I also hope you can look past the hilarity to recognize what a ridiculous thought process this really was. I hope my answer now, as a fitness professional, will perhaps shed some light toward the steps that are necessary to initiate positive changes. The word "*toned*" simply means holding onto muscle tissue at the very least, or increasing it slightly, while simultaneously losing body fat that is most likely concealing the muscle tone. Now, this may sound simplistic; and it *is* in theory. Getting "*toned*" is not the real challenge. The real challenge for most of us is finding an *effective* program that works!

Getting There...From Here

Our bodies begin to look more defined by building just a little more muscle and losing excessive fat that normally conceals the muscle. Not to worry, ladies — you will not morph into a "muscle-bound" bodybuilder overnight. It's not genetically possible. It's really not possible, so please put any fears to rest. Also, the muscle-building process is a slow one; so you are always in complete control of how you'd like to change your body. The muscle you develop will appear feminine and shapely, giving you that toned look that you so desire. By putting the training methods outlined throughout *The Power of Champions* into practice and becoming more educated about how to implement *effective* aerobic exercise to burn body fat, you have all the synergistic elements in place to achieve your goals. As a result, your moderate aerobic exercise will become more effective in helping you burn excess body fat. Not only will you burn fat while you exercise, but by building a little more muscle, you will now be burning fat all day — while you eat, while you watch TV, even while you sleep. That is the power of Synergy, and the secret to getting "*toned*."

More is Not Always Better

Helen was the ideal client. She was ideal because she came to me with an open mind. She also recognized that her current program was no longer working. Helen never had a problem with her weight - until she reached her 50's. As we reviewed her history, it was obvious why she was having problems now; she spent years as either a chronic dieter or ignoring her nutritional needs.

Existing on a somewhat modified "low-carb" diet, Helen was basically starving herself and depleting her energy reserves with a lack of carbohydrates — the body's preferential fuel source. She had been working out diligently, maybe even with a little too much vengeance. She needed to pull the reigns in.

What was happening here was a classic case of under eating/over training. Consequently, Helen's metabolism had come to a grinding halt causing the plateau and her frustration. She was working unbelievably hard and not getting anywhere. Helen's calories were way too low for her energy demands. At the training studio, we took the time to discuss the importance of supportive nutrition in relation to Synergy. If you don't provide your body with the raw material it needs, it will not be capable of muscle building and repair and will break down muscle tissue for energy, while holding on to body fat stores for security. Translated to mean; without a doubt, you will get nowhere.

This story does have a happy ending. Helen applied the principles of Synergy, started to see the changes, and was elated! Every time she walked through the door, her body was becoming more compact and streamlined. She went from a size 12 dress down to a size 8 in no time at all! Helen literally is one of my best advertisements to this very day because she took the time to get educated. Her education paid off big time — not only in her new shape, but also in her enthusiasm and zest for life! Would you have ever thought that exercising *less,* and eating *more,* would be the key?

A Toned Body *Needs* Synergy!

Remember ladies, it is always the *combination* of principles that work together harmoniously, which will yield optimal results. Moderate aerobic exercise burns body fat, strength training builds lean muscle, and supportive nutrition fuels the body and boosts metabolism. Once you begin to understand and embrace these concepts, a body that is both lean and strong as well as energetic and flexible will be yours. In short, a body that is *toned.*

You make the decision to become empowered when you abandon the notion that the secret to long-term weight loss lies in any one technology. Real work is involved but with that work comes real *results* that can be quite astounding! You may never again look to another fashion magazine, the New York Times Best-Sellers List, or your friends and neighbors for weight-loss solutions again. I *didn't. . .* now, they come to *me!*

Karen Webster, ACE, AAAI

The Body Works Studio
Heritage Center
3326 Old York Road
Suite B105
Furlong, PA 18925
215-794-0372
Karen.Webster@thepowerofchampions.com

Specialization for Women's Issues by Angela Ursprung

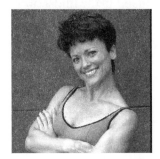

Champion Angela Ursprung of Raleigh, North Carolina, *The Body Sculptress*, brings experience, immense compassion and a profound belief in people's ability to overcome life's challenges in providing the groundwork for helping thousands of women sculpt bodies that are better than they ever dreamed possible!

After spending many years working primarily with women, I've learned that as a gender we have a lot of issues that need to be factored in when it comes to sculpting a leaner, healthier body — body type, busy lifestyle, menstruation, menopause, fibromyalgia and other chronic issues, not to mention food!

Some women tend to carry their body fat all over their bodies (an apple) while others tend to carry it mainly in their hips and thighs (a pear). As I am an apple myself, I've always been rather envious of those who can quickly develop beautifully sculpted abs, arms and backs while covering the higher fat areas of your lower body. Apples, on the other hand, have to lose their body fat everywhere in order for any one body part to appear lean and sculpted.

Additionally, while some of us tend to be naturally athletic with the ability to quickly gain and lose muscle and fat (mesomorph), others of us have a real difficult time gaining muscle (ectomorph) or a very difficult time losing body fat (endomorph). In Champion Bryan Lanham's chapter, 'Sizing Up Exercise: Training Different Body Types with Different Routines,' you can determine your body type and how to design your individual program accordingly.

Adding to the body type issues are the life issues. The chief concern among many women is the inability to find time for themselves while caring for a spouse, children, aging parents, career, committees, and church and neighborhood obligations. I often hear, "But I'm too busy to exercise," and in some cases it really is true.

Regardless of what is going on and how important each commitment seems to be, how vital would it be if you suddenly found yourself with a chronic or fatal condition? It is paramount that you make the time for your health—20 to 30 minutes most days is a good place to start.

Then factor in our body's monthly battle for our will! Many of us stay on track rather well for three weeks only to find ourselves back at ground zero during one emotionally-laden chocolate and ice cream festival. What's my secret? I don't bring temptations into the house! Remember, if it's not good for you, it's not good for your family either. Don't feel guilty. Feel empowered!

Here's some good news…menstruation affects exercise! Exercising after ovulation at the midpoint of the menstrual cycle is easier and burns more fat than exercising in the first week of the menstrual cycle. So plan to really burn it up during the midpoint to make bigger fat-burn gains!

Perhaps you have been blessed by the ending of your war's battle, only to find yourself in the midst of another very similar onslaught. You are suddenly unable to control your body temperature, your sexual drive, your menstrual cycles, and your emotions as your hormones rise and fall at a rate that you can neither anticipate nor control. Worse still is the fact that you have to deal with this as a sleep-deprived zombie!

Like menstruation, the trick is to work hardest when you have energy in order to make big gains and counteract those days when you feel weak and lethargic. Exercise, proper nutrition and rest will help you minimize the negative effects of this transition.

It is usually during this same time that I hear women starting to use the dreaded words…fibromyalgia and arthritis. Often, we are suddenly held captive by a body which experiences ongoing chronic pain that is confusing and may seem to get worse with exercise rather than better.

We are also suddenly held accountable for poor posture and repetitive-type motions that we have perhaps done for our entire lives. For example, if you have been lifting improperly for 20 years, you may find that you have lower back and knee injuries. If you have been carrying a heavy briefcase in your right hand for 20 years, you may find that you have tendonitis in your right shoulder and/or forearm. And if you have been driving the kids around and eating at fast food drive-thrus for 20 years, you may find that you are dealing with osteoporosis or an autoimmune deficiency caused by inadequate nutrition. For these chronic ailments, you are well advised to seek the counsel of an expert prior to beginning any exercise program. Remember, your best bet is to start a healthy lifestyle before you develop any issues!

Finally, we must address the fact that as we slow down with career, family and wildly-fluctuating hormones, our bodies begin to accumulate body fat as quickly as our pain and anguish seem to build. This means more body fat, more self-doubt, and a higher risk of disease to name a few consequences.

So what do we do? We start a diet. Did it ever occur to you that the root of the word diet is "die?" The real problem with diets is that there is a grain of truth to each one which may provide you some sort of progress for a short length of time, but the diet always ends. When the diet ends, your body fat percentage increases as your lean mass (muscle and bone) decreases.

Generally speaking at this point most of us decide to try the old diet again or perhaps a new diet—the new "thing" and the cycle repeats itself. And what happens? The diet works for a while, then the diet ends, and the body wastes once more. Every single time this yo-yo effect occurs your lean mass is less and less able to recover. That means that your metabolism takes hit after hit and as time goes on, it drops dramatically.

So what is a woman to do? There are as many combinations of variables as there are women in the world, so no one program will work perfectly for everyone, but this one will give you a nice baseline to begin with. As you get stronger or decide you want something different, consider contacting me on the Internet.

It is a program that all women can use to fight the negative effects of body type, lifestyle, hormonal onslaught, and chronic ailments. The best health and fitness program is going to incorporate strength training that works every single muscle in your body. I've included "compound" exercises — exercises that work more than one body part at a time, thereby providing maximal benefit while saving time.

Additionally, a good program will include activity to condition your heart and lungs. Anything that is done over a period of 15-60 minutes that you enjoy and that causes you to have to breathe hard is a good starting point.

Stretching is another component of a good program as your connective tissue, spinal column and muscles need to move through their full range of motion in order to achieve optimal health. Plenty of clean, filtered water, a good multivitamin, a women's formula, and calcium should be included.

Do your very best to minimize your reliance on processed food in favor of natural food. Fresh fruits and vegetables, whole grains, seeds and nuts, dairy, fresh and natural meats and fish are all recommended. Section 6, 'Eat Like a Champion,' offers practical advice that you can begin implementing today for a nutritional approach that is synergistic with your fitness program.

Lastly, and perhaps less apparent, is the requirement that you believe that you are worthy and deserving of spending time, energy and money on yourself—not your kids, not your spouse, not your parents, but on and for yourself. You must be able to make yourself a priority or you aren't going to get to ride the health train. It's that simple.

Here's a sample program to get your started. Each/most weekdays:

6:00 am -

- Awake
- 1-2 glasses of filtered water
- 5-15 minutes of planning and meditation
- Strength - 10 jump jacks*, pushups, superman, crunches, sit-stands**, chair dips, lunges, and overhead press
- Shower

    * can be low intensity for those with bad knees
    ** find a straight back chair; sit down, stand up; repeat

7:00 am – Breakfast; 1 water

10:00 am – Snack; 1 water

12:00 pm – Lunch; 1 water

3:00 pm – Snack; 1 water

6:00 pm – Dinner; 1 water

7:30 pm -

- Cardio - 15-60 minutes, e.g., walk, bike, run, elliptical trainer, jump rope, swim, climb stairs, etc.
- Stretch - perform at least 1 stretch for each muscle group and hold it for 20-30 seconds
- drink 2-3 glasses of water

Repeat the exercise cycle 1-3 times.

Angela Ursprung, MBA, ACSM

Angela.Ursprung@thepowerofchampions.com
www.thebodysculptress.com

Reducing and Shaping Your Hips and Thighs by Darrell Morris

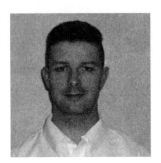

Champion Darrell Morris of Denver, Colorado works with all age groups interested in learning how to stay and/or get fit for life. Helping people feel good and gain confidence that they can achieve their goals is a true passion!

Do you want your hips and thighs to look like those you see on magazine covers or your favorite athlete or movie actress?

Are you ready to take action to reduce and shape your hips and thighs? I'm going to assume that your answer is a resounding "Yes!"

First, I need you to free your mind of all the current and past exercises you have done to achieve this elusive goal. Clear the slate. Each day I see exercisers doing every imaginable exercise to reduce and shape these areas and I often stop to ask, "Why are you doing that exercise?" Overwhelmingly the response is, "I want to work on this area right here" as they point to their hips and thighs. More often than not, they are using the hip abductor machine followed by the adductor machine, or vice versa. Unfortunately, those machines are ill equipped to effectively work those areas to which they have pointed. In my opinion, the only reason those two machines are in the gym is because they 'sell' memberships.

Appropriate exercise selection will train the musculature as a whole rather than with isolation movements. To do so, you need to incorporate exercises that will challenge all the muscles - both stabilizers and prime movers. The prime movers are the muscles that you are probably most familiar with - hamstrings, quadriceps, adductors and glutes. The stabilizers are the abductors and hip external rotators. Primary exercises are those that work the entire hip and thigh area. Secondary exercises isolate a particular muscle group.

Your body functions in several directions - sideways, forward, backward and twisting. Selecting exercises that target all the musculature that can be performed in a variety of directions is ideal.

The primary exercises will be your dominant exercises because they effectively train the entire hip and thigh region. Before we move on, there is a point that needs to be driven home here - you cannot spot reduce! Simply because you are moving your quadriceps, for example, doesn't mean that the energy is coming from that area. It comes from the most accessible area at the time of your movement. So if the triceps have readily available calories to burn while you are performing a lunge, that's where the energy comes from. This supports the synergistic formula - aerobic activity, a concern for muscle and proper nutrition - which are all necessary to achieve your health and fitness goals. Performing these exercises will help to strengthen and shape the muscles worked. The other synergistic elements help to reduce body fat which shows off those toned muscles. For more on the benefits of strength training and reducing body fat, be sure to read Champion Peter Piranio's chapter entitled 'A Concern for Muscle' and Champion Amy Powlison's chapter on 'Fat Loss Rather than a Focus on Pounds.'

The Primary Exercises

Lunges and squats are the two most basic compound movements that will shape the hips and thighs. These exercises mimic our daily activities and help us become more efficient as a result. Here are some key points to help you perform the lunge and squat both safely and effectively.

Lunge

- From a standing position with good posture draw your belly button in toward your spine (do not suck in the abs); feet should be shoulder width apart with toes pointed forward
- Step forward with your right foot and descend slowly by bending at the hips, knees and ankles; hips and knees should be at a 90° angle at the bottom of the range of motion
- Maintain the weight of the forward foot between the mid-foot and heel
- The knee should track between your 1st and 2nd toe; you should be able to see your toes at all times during this exercise
- Perform the downward reps slowly and concentrate on the descent while maintaining your posture and keeping your torso erect
- When you have completed the lunges on the right side, repeat on the left

Squat

- Start with feet shoulder width apart; draw your belly button toward the spine (do not suck in the abs)
- Descend slowly by bending at the knees and hips
- While descending maintain weight between the mid-foot and heel
- During the ascent drive through the feet with the weight evenly distributed between the mid-foot and heel
- The knee should track over the 2nd and 3rd toes; you should be able to see your toes at all times during this exercise
- Perform the descent slowly and concentrate
- Descend as far as you can with control; if necessary, start with partial squats and progress to full squats over time

Practice in front of a mirror to be sure your form is correct. Mastering the basics of the squat and lunge will allow you to take on the many variations of both exercises with confidence and continued results.

The secondary exercises allow you to isolate a particular muscle group of the hips or thighs. Here are a few of the secondary exercises that have helped my clients achieve success.

Muscle Group	Exercise
Quadriceps (front of thigh)	Seated Leg Extension
	Single Leg Seated Extension
	Single Leg Standing Extension
Hamstrings (back of thigh)	Seated/Prone Leg Curl
	Supine Ball Curl
	Standing Single Leg Curl
	Straight Leg Deadlift
Glutes (buttocks)	Standing Hip Extension
	Donkey Kick
Adductors (inner thigh)	Standing Cable Adduction
Abductors (outer thigh)	Standing Cable Abduction

Now I am sure you are thinking that I missed some of your favorites. There are so many variations but I can tell you these are the exercises that I know work!

So how do you choose which exercises you should perform? Let's make it simple! When you design your program, choose one exercise from the primary list and one from the secondary list. Variation is the key to getting and keeping shapely hips and thighs. Your body is designed for movement and the majority of that movement is created in the hips and thighs. Experiment with different combinations. Here are a few to get you started.

Squat/Leg Extension	Lunge/Straight Leg Deadlift
Lunge/Seated Hamstring Curl	Squat/Supine Hamstring Curl w/stability ball
Squat/Hip Extension	Lunge/Standing Leg Extension

Listen to your body. If you experience pain, it is a sign that something is wrong. Do not work through the pain. Check your form carefully and, if correct, seek the advice of your healthcare provider. Otherwise, you are setting yourself up for injury. Champion Erik Naclerio offers good advice for preventing injuries in his chapter, 'Injury Free Resistance Training.'

You have probably noticed that I have not said a word about repetitions, sets, weights, or how often you should perform any of the above exercises. I have my reasons. The exercises were chosen to fit in the training cycles. Where you are in the training cycle and your fitness level will determine how many repetitions and sets, how much weight and how often you should perform these exercises. I will tell you this much though … always start light and make sure you are doing the exercise correctly before progressing.

Darrell Morris, B.A., NSCA CPT, NASM PES

RR Personal Training
303-584-0940 Studio
720-298-0281 Cell
Darrell.Morris@thepowerofchampions.com

SECTION ELEVEN
Options for Champions

Notes from Phil

We've arrived at the final section of the book, and as I'm sure you recognize by now, this is not an ending, but a beginning. You should be well on your way to physical excellence and, with the knowledge you've acquired, the obstacles are fewer. You're gaining mastery of your mind, your attitude, your body, and your performance, and you're moving forward toward the achievement of your most driving physical goals.

In The Power of Champions, *we've discussed "needs." The primary necessities that allow for positive physical change are the right nutrition, moderate aerobic exercise, a concern for muscle, the right attitude, follow-through, and downtime. Beyond the needs, there are options. There are almost 20,000 commercial health clubs in the United States and somewhere in the vicinity of half a million individuals carrying business cards that read "Personal Trainer." You don't "need" a health club, nor do you "need" a trainer, but there are absolute virtues to recognizing the potential intrinsic values of these options.*

We'll conclude with a section in which Champion Joe Stankowski helps you decide whether a health club is a wise option for you and Champion Vickie Burnham shares a perspective on Personal Training.

As you complete this section, I want you to feel a sense of achievement. You've completed a process of empowerment and now the sky's the limit. You can take your physical improvement to levels you might never even have dreamed of. For some of you, competition may be in your future, for others you may simply relish in the joy that you have a new vitality and energy allowing you to become a more productive member of the workforce or of your family. The Power of Champions *should serve as a reference you'll pull from the shelf again and again to find new inspiration and renewed motivation. You've had the privilege of learning from more than 50 of the world's top fitness professionals, and we're all here, in your corner, prompting you to succeed.*

Congratulations on making an investment in your own betterment, and enjoy the journey! Time to consider your options as you read the section entitled, "Options for Champions."

Is A Health Club Right For Me? by Joe Stankowski

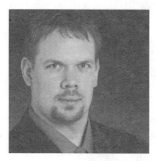

Champion Joe Stankowski of Wilmington, Delaware owns AbsoluteFitnessUSA.com. He also guides clients to success in the comfort and convenience of their homes and outdoors. Joe is the Official Fitness Trainer for MISS DELAWARE USA®.

No citizen has the right to be an amateur in the matter of physical training.

What a disgrace it is for a man to grow old without ever seeing

the beauty and strength of which his body is capable.

- Socrates 469-399 B.C.

While the question 'Is A Health Club Right for Me?' may seem like a straightforward one, you are about to learn why it is practically impossible for me to give you a simple 'yes' or 'no' answer. I firmly believe that you are the person that needs to make this decision. I also know that you'll make the best choice when armed with the information in this chapter.

Rather than suggest you jump blindly into a gym membership that you may not need, you might be shocked to read what I'm about to say...

Nobody actually NEEDS a health club.

Now why would a fitness professional make a statement like that? You may want to exercise at a health club or even think you should. The basic fact is that health clubs simply offer a collection of equipment, which can be used to improve one's fitness. This alone doesn't necessarily make it the best option. But don't rush out to cancel your membership just yet either!

For the record – while I typically work with my clients in their own homes or outdoors, I am in no way "anti-gym." In fact, commercial gyms have long been an important part of my own training and I expect they will always continue to be as long as I have a pulse! I even recommend them to people who I feel can benefit from them. But if you want to know the whole story, please read on.

According to the International Health, Racquet and Sports Association (IHRSA), there were barely 6,000 health clubs in the U.S. in 1982. In 2003, there were over 20,200. More than 36 million Americans belong to a health club. Yearly total industry revenues exceed $13 billion. Regular attendance has nearly tripled since 1987. By the sound of things, you'd expect America to be in great physical shape.

Figures from the U.S. Center for Disease Control conjure up a much more disturbing image. In America, 64% of adults are overweight or obese. Fifteen percent of children ages 6-19 are also considered overweight. Along with these figures, throughout the 1990's, diabetes increased 33% across the nation. And much of the world is following in our super-sized footsteps.

Opportunity for healthy activity is all around. I'm not aware of any city, town, or even the smallest neighborhood that doesn't provide at least the basic ingredients for daily activity. There are personal trainers that come to you and private training studios everywhere. Home equipment can be an affordable and effective option when used as part of a complete program. Parks frequently have walking trails, bike paths, and tennis courts. The list goes on and on...

Even though the "success" rate is debatable, I have no doubt that health clubs are here to stay. In addition to the national chains and local gyms, you can find community or church-based exercise programs. Many corporations and residential developments now offer fitness facilities. Since the late 1800's, YMCA facilities around the world started adding gyms, swimming pools and bowling alleys to their boarding houses. (Did you know racquetball and basketball originated in Y's?) Today, there are over 2400 YMCA facilities throughout the United States offering a variety of exercise options.

So what gives? It appears to me that health clubs fail to incorporate the one essential element that virtually guarantees success. It's a well know "secret" among fitness professionals and I promise to let you know exactly what it is!

To make the most appropriate decision when considering your fitness options, you must first answer these six questions:

What is my goal? As you more clearly describe your goals, you increase the likelihood you'll achieve them. Accurately define your purpose in training. Can a health club support these goals? For tips and strategies on setting goals, see Champion Tony Rodriguez's chapter, 'Be Your Own "Fitness Coach".'

What do I enjoy? If you dread something, no matter how "good" it may be, how long do you really think you'll stick with it? Would you enjoy training at a gym?

Do I prefer to exercise alone or with others? If you prefer to workout by yourself but can't get to the gym outside of peak times, a health club may not be what you're looking for. But if a social setting is just as important to you as realizing your fitness goals, a health club membership may be a good choice for you.

What happens if my priorities change? Unfortunately, a majority of people who join gyms don't stick with it past the first 6 to 8 weeks. Will you still have to pay for a membership you're not using? Can one health club offer everything you need, even if your goals change along the way?

Will it work? Are there systems in place to help you achieve your goals? Fitness training is not one-size-fits-all. Do you know if you're following the appropriate plan?

Do you have a true understanding of what it takes to achieve your fitness goals? As much as I may enjoy tinkering around with my car, when it comes down to it, I need reliable transportation right now! Because this is very important to me, I have no problem paying a trained mechanic to do the job right the first time. If you're not a "do-it-yourselfer" and your fitness goals are serious business, personal trainers are the expert technicians when it comes to fitness.

If you're considering hiring a personal trainer but don't know where to start, visit www.thepowerofchampions.com where you will find a special report explaining the most important questions you need to ask.

To fully appreciate the value of a health club, you should also consider potential drawbacks:

- Inconvenient location
- Potential distractions (e.g., loud music or the girl wearing spandex!)
- Intimidating setting (real or perceived)
- Long-term, no-escape contracts
- Often overcrowded during peak hours
- Sometimes lack experienced, personal instruction

While statistics suggest that more people are beginning to recognize the value of gyms, you must understand that spending a couple of hours in the gym each week is not enough. A health club membership should be viewed as a just one component of a healthy lifestyle. One of the most important messages I try to convey to my clients is that a workout alone will never produce the changes they're looking for.

So when it comes down to it, all you really need is:

- Specific goal(s)
- A plan for success
- A system to monitor progress

Most importantly, the "secret ingredient" I mentioned earlier. Ok, ok. I know I promised to tell you the one element health clubs can never provide. It's not a new machine or fitness class. And it's definitely not another "miracle" diet pill.

You probably won't believe how simple this secret really is. No matter how well equipped a gym may be, all the reading, planning and talking in the world won't do you a bit of good until you consciously choose to take _ACTION_. Unless you commit to the ongoing process of an active and healthy lifestyle, both in and out of the gym, you will likely be disappointed with your progress.

So lose the excuses and move your body!

Now you have solid information to help you make the best decision for you. If you have well-defined **goals**, motivation to **act** and a **plan** for success, you *might* find a health club to be an invaluable piece of your fitness puzzle.

Now you should be able to answer the question – Is a health club right for me?

Joe Stankowski, ACE, NASM CPT, IDEA Master Trainer

302-898-8373
Joe.Stankowski@thepowerofchampions.com
www.AbsoluteFitnessUSA.com
www.PageantryFitness.com

Personal Training is "Personal" by Vickie Burnham

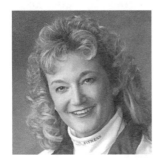

Champion Vickie Burnham of Bangor, Maine owns Innovative Fitness where she offers her clients the highest level of quality, personalized fitness training with comprehensive programs that include cardiovascular, flexibility and strength resistance training, nutrition counseling, sports performance camps and yoga.

Barbara Francis had been diagnosed with Rheumatoid Arthritis (RA) several years before becoming a client of Innovative Fitness in September of 1998.

Barbara always thought RA was a joint disease that grandparents have, but soon found out that this is not the case. She was placed on painkillers and steroids like Percocet, Darvan, Arava, and other drugs, but none had an effect on her pain. After the first year, she began chemotherapy injections of Methotrexate to help boost her immune system to keep the disease at bay. By this time she had gained a lot of weight and was so debilitated that she was almost totally dependent on her husband. She could not dress herself, comb her own hair or continue her passion for making Native American basketry due to the pain and immobility. "People started expressing pity for my plight and I became very angry," Barbara states.

Barbara describes the disease best as an autoimmune disease that aids in the destruction of healthy bone. In addition, the "good" and "bad" days of living with this disease can create havoc with one's emotions. The technical description is best summarized as the inflammation of the lining of many different joints in the body. This inflammation can cause a lot of pain, stiffness, swelling, warmth, and redness. The affected joints may also lose their shape, which can constrict their normal movement. The disease is known to have flare ups in its active stages but can also have remissions where there will be little or no symptoms. As with Barbara, RA can also affect other parts of the body, including the blood, the lungs, and the heart. However, researchers now believe that treating the disease early and aggressively may not only control the joint pain, inflammation, and stiffness, but may also slow the progression of the disease.

At the age of 42, Barbara made a decision to take her life back. She obtained medical clearance from her rheumatologist and began searching for a gym that provided personal training. Aside from the fact that she had not been in a gym since high school, Barbara felt very strongly about approaching exercise in a manner that would keep her injury free. That is when she entered into a partnership training agreement with Innovative Fitness.

Since then, the outcome has been remarkable. Over time, Barbara started dressing herself, engaging in social events, and most of all, she revisited her passion for basket making. She has won several awards for her baskets all over the United States, including a first place ribbon at the Santa Fe Indian Market in New Mexico. A documentary film in her honor was made which has also won awards. Most recently she spent three weeks touring the states for the Smithsonian Institute doing research on the history of Native American Culture.

Barbara has a history of panic attacks when in crowds and a major fear of flying. With both of these issues now very much under control, Barbara attributes exercise to breaking through these barriers. As she gained the ability to physically do more on her own, she continued to gain confidence in herself. "I have been in situations where my trainer's words will come back to me. Last time I was on a plane, I could hear her telling me 'Breathe, Barbara, breathe,' and this helped me stay focused and more relaxed. Concentrated breathing has also been helpful to me in several medical situations."

In addition to regaining control of her life and hobbies, Barbara has reduced the medications needed to manage the pain and attacks brought on by RA. Her physicians attribute her success of managing this disease and accomplishments in pain control to her exercise regimen, integrity, and determination.

I have written this chapter to express to people that everyone has their own reasons for exercising, and every client's programming needs to be based on the individual. There is no cookie cutter or blanket approach to personal training. A vast majority of gym members exercise to lose those unwanted pounds. However, clients come to a certified personal trainer with more specific goals, e.g., injury prevention, pain management through exercise, guided rehabilitation after a cardiac event, or even powerlifting. They are all very personal. In Barbara's case, there were many variables to prepare for and obstacles to overcome.

Barbara's exercise appointments had to be scheduled around the unpredictability of flare-ups, sleepless nights, joint inflammation, and physical pain. Inability to plan ahead because of these situations was frustrating for Barbara. A lot of trainer/client dialogue was needed to observe if the symptoms were related to certain activities or from physical or emotional stressors. Working with her nutrition, ensuring appropriate rest, planning exercise around her injections, or having medication adjusted by her physician would usually help overcome these obstacles. Additionally, because Barbara's immune system is constantly at a deficit, she is very susceptible to any contagious viruses that are hovering around the gym. Communication was crucial at times to determine if it was wise for her to enter the gym on certain days. We always had a Plan B or even Plan C in place to deal with these situations so Barbara would not feel like she was falling behind.

In order to increase Barbara's stamina, an endurance-based strength training program was implemented. This was a challenge because the RA had damaged her lungs. She had to learn how to breathe deeply enough to help improve the delivery of oxygen to her muscles. Resistance started out as simply as pushing one hand against the other. These types of isometric exercises proved to be very beneficial in Barbara's exercise program in that they gave her the best results in the least amount of time. "Now don't think it was a walk in the park," Barbara jokes. "I thought dying would be more humane some days after I had finished in the gym."

Muscle flexibility and joint mobility has been essential in order to regain and retain as much normal motion as possible. It has also been the key to improving the quality of her joint movements. Her warm up included full body stretching, as well as both active and passive range of motion joint exercises.

The fame that comes with Barbara's talent in basket making does not come without a price. When Barbara travels as an artist, we work on relaxation techniques and exercises she can do on the road prior to her departure. Upon her return we work to "undo" the rigors of the trip. As one might imagine, this is not always a simple process.

Over time Barbara was able to move on to more power-based exercises using a progressive, graded, and systematic approach to getting stronger…and she definitely was getting stronger! Here was a woman who at one time could not tie her own shoes and is now pressing over 500 pounds on the hip sled. Barbara remembers when "Ten crunches killed me, but at the end of six months it was three sets of 12, and now 100 crunches seem easy." Remember, however, this level of improvement and achievement has evolved over months and years of hard work with carefully planned programs and teamwork.

Seven years ago, Barbara knew her prognosis was not good unless she took control of her body and her disease. Barbara has a tremendous attitude, a ton of self-discipline, and a personal trainer that takes the time to clearly set up a program personal to her needs. Getting back to Champion Jonathan Ross' article, 'Excellence - A Culmination of Tiny Steps,' at the beginning of *The Power of Champions*, Barbara exemplifies the principle that the right attitude can move mountains - and change a life forever!

Vickie Burnham, ACE

Innovative Fitness
366 Griffin Road
Bangor, ME 04401
207-942-3200
Vickie.Burnham@thepowerofchampions.com

References

Balancing Body, Mind and Spirit by Champion Michelle Hazlewood

[1] Excerpted from 'Maps to Ecstasy' by Gabrielle Roth. Used with permission from New World Library, Novato, CA 94949, www.newworldlibrary.com.

Fat Loss Rather than a Focus on Pounds by Champion Amy Powlison

[2] Cotton, Richard T., ed. <u>Personal Trainer Manual</u>. San Diego, CA: American Council on Exercise, 1996.

Measuring Body Composition Effectively by Champion Lisa Martin

Baechle, T.R. and R.W. Earle. <u>Essentials of Strength and Conditioning</u>, 2nd edition. Champaign, IL: Human Kinetics, 2000.

Bloomquist, Michele. "Getting Rid of Cellulite." WebMD. 2000. http://my.webmd.com/content/article/13/1689_50311.htm?lastselectedguid={5FE84E90-BC77-4056-A91C-9531713CA348}.

[3] Cotton, Richard T., ed. <u>Personal Trainer Manual</u>. San Diego, CA: American Council on Exercise, 1996.

Escott-Stump, Sylvia and L. Kathleen Mahan. <u>Krause's Food, Nutrition & Diet Therapy</u>, 10th edition. Philadelphia, PA: W.B. Saunders Company, 2000.

Groff, James L. and Sareen S. Gropper. <u>Advanced Nutrition and Human Metabolism</u>, 3rd edition. Belmont, CA: Wadsworth/Thomson Learning, 2000.

Lee, Robert D. and David C. Nieman. <u>Nutritional Assessment</u>, 2nd edition. St. Louis, MO: McGraw-Hill Companies, 1996.

Sharkey, Brian J. <u>Fitness and Health</u>, 4th edition. Champaign, IL: Human Kinetics, 1997.

The Other Benefits of Exercise by Champion Jason T. Hoffman

[4] Pate, R.R., M.L. Small, J.G. Ross, J.C. Young, K.H. Flint and C.W. Warren. "School physical education." Journal of School Health 65(8) (1995): 339-343 EJ 520 865.

[5] Katz, Warren A., M.D., and Carl Sherman. "Exercise for Osteoporosis." <u>The Physician and Sports Medicine</u> Vol. 26, No. 2 (1998, February).

[6] Coyle, E. F. "Cardiovascular function during exercise: neural control factors." <u>Sports Science Exchange</u> Vol. 4 (1991, September): 34.

[7] Skrinar, G., K. V. Unger, and D. S. Hutchinson. "Effects of exercise training in young adults with psychiatric disabilities." <u>Canadian Journal of Rehabilitation</u> Vol. 5 (1992): 151-157.

[8] Wilson, R.S., D.A. Bennett, J.L. Bienias, et al. "Cognitive activity and incident AD in a population-based sample of older persons." Neurology Vol. 59 (2002): 1910-1914.

[9] Stefanick, M. L., S. Mackey, et al. "Effects of diet and exercise in men and postmenopausal women with low levels of HDL cholesterol and high levels of LDL cholesterol." New England Journal of Medicine Vol. 399(1) (1998): 12-20.

[10] Whelton, A., X. Chin, X. "Effect of aerobic exercise on blood pressure: a meta-analysis of randomized, controlled trials." SP. Annals of Internal Medicine Vol. 136 (2002): 493-503.

Injury Free Resistance Training by Champion Erik Naclerio

[11] Prentica, W. E. "Flexibility: Roundtable." NSCA Journal 6(4) (1984): 10-22, 71-73.

[12] Baechle, T.R. and R.W. Earle. Essentials of Strength and Conditioning, 2nd edition. Champaign, IL: Human Kinetics, 2000.

[13] Totten, L. "Kneewraps." NSCA Journal 12(5) (1990): 36-38.

[14] Chaffin, D.B. and G. Anderson. Occupational Biomechanics. New York: McGraw-Hill.1986

[15] Bartelik, D.L. "The Role of Abdominal Pressure in Relieving the Pressure on the Lumbar Intervertebral Discs." Journal of Bone and Joint Surgery 398(4) (1957): 718-725.

[16] Morris, J.M., D.B. Lucas and B. Bresler. "Role of the Trunk in Stability of the Spine." Journal of Bone and Joint Surgery 43A (1961): 327-351.

[17] Wallack, R.M. "Big League Shoulder Protection." Men's Fitness. Weider Publications.

Finding the Athlete Inside by David Thomas

Advanced Program Design: A Chek Institute Video Correspondence Series. South Vulcan Avenue Suite 101, San Diego, CA. 1999.

Chek, Paul. Should Athletes Train Like Bodybuilders. San Diego CA: A Chek Institute Publication, 2000.

Baechle, T.R. and R.W. Earle. Essentials of Strength and Conditioning, 2nd edition. Champaign, IL: Human Kinetics, 2000.

The Routine that Worked Wonders by Champion Stephen Holt

Lee, Diane. The Pelvic Girdle: An Approach to the Examination and Treatment of the Lumbo-Pelvic-Hip Region, 2nd edition. Churchill Livingstone. New York, 1999.

Vleeming, Andry, ed. Movement, Stability and Low Back Pain: The Essential Role of the Pelvis. New York, NY: Churchill Livingstone, 1997.

Myers, Thomas. <u>The Anatomy Trains: Myofascial Meridians for Manual and Movement Therapies</u>. New York, NY: Churchill Livingstone, 2001.

Periodization **by Champion Brian Schiff**

[18] Matveyev, L.P. <u>Periodization of Sports Training</u>. Moscow: Fiscultura i Sport, 1966.

[19] Baechle, T.R. and R.W. Earle. <u>Essentials of Strength and Conditioning</u>, 2nd edition. Champaign, IL: Human Kinetics, 2000.

[20] Stone, M.H., H.S. O'Bryant, and J. Garhammer. "A hypothetical model for strength training." <u>Journal of Sports Medicine and Physical Fitness</u> 21 (1981): 336, 342-351.

[21] Komi, P.V. "Training of muscle strength and power: Introduction of neuromotoric, hypertrophic and mechanical factors." <u>International Journal of Sports Medicine</u> 7(suppl) (1986): 101-105.

Putting Your Heart into Your Exercise Program **by Champion Brett A. Pruitt**

American College of Sports Medicine. <u>ACSM Fitness Book</u>, 3rd edition. Champaign, IL: Human Kinetics, 2003.

American College of Sports Medicine. <u>ACSM's Guidelines for Exercise Testing and Prescription</u>, 6th edition. Philadelphia, PA: Lippincott, Williams & Wilkins, 2000.

Strength Training and Blood Pressure: The Heart of the Matter **by Champion Wayne Westcott**

[22] Westcott, W. and Baechle, T. <u>Strength Training for Seniors</u>. Champaign, IL: Human Kinetics, 1999.

[23] Blumenthal, J., W. Siegel, and M. Appelbaum. "Failure of exercise to reduce blood pressure in patients with hypertension." <u>Journal of the American Medical Association</u> 266 (1991): 2098-2101.

[24] Smutok, M., C. Reece, P. Kokkinos, et al. "Aerobics vs. strength training for risk factor intervention in middle-aged men at high risk for coronary heart disease." <u>Metabolism</u> 42 (1993): 177-184.

[25] Harris, K. and R. Holly. "Physiological response to circuit weight training in borderline hypertensive subjects." <u>Medicine and Science in Sports and Exercise</u> 10 (1987): 246-252.

[26] Kelly, G. "Dynamic resistance exercise and resting blood pressure in healthy adults: a meta-analysis." <u>Journal of Applied Physiology</u> 82 (1997): 1559-1565.

[27] Westcott, W. and B. Howes. "Blood pressure response during weight training exercise." <u>National Strength and Conditioning Association Journal</u> 5 (1983): 67-71.

[28] American College of Sports Medicine. <u>Guidelines for Exercise Testing and Prescription</u>. Philadelphia, PA: Lea and Febiger, 1991.

[29] Westcott, W. "Strength training and blood pressure." <u>American Fitness Quarterly</u> 5 (1986): 38-39.

[30] Westcott, W. <u>Strength Fitness: Physiological Principles and Training Techniques</u>, 4th edition. Duluque, IA: William C. Brown/McGraw-Hill, 1995.

[31] Westcott, W. and M. Pappas. "Immediate effects of circuit strength training on blood pressure." <u>American Fitness Quarterly</u> 6 (1987): 43-44.

[32] Westcott, W. "Blood Pressure response to strength training." <u>Perspective</u> 28 (2002): 26-28.

[33] Westcott, W. and J. Guy. "A physical evolution: Sedentary adults see marked improvements from training as little as two days a week." <u>IDEA Today</u> 14 (1996): 58-65.

[34] Westcott, W., F. Dolan and T. Cavicchi. "Golf and strength training are compatible activities." <u>Journal of Strength and Conditioning</u>, 18 (1996): 54-56.

The Benefits of Frequent Eating by Champion Billy Beck III

[35] Amaha, E. "Gripping times." Far Eastern Economic Review 162 (1999): 38-40. UMI-ProQuest Direct. [Online] [April 13, 1999].

[35] Nishizawa, T., I. Akaoka, Y. Nishida, Y. Kawaguchi, E. Hayashi, and T. Yashimura. "Some factor related to obesity in the Japanese sumo wrestler." <u>The American Journal of Clinical Nutrition</u> 29 (1976): 1167-1174.

[36] Amaha, E. "Gripping times." Far Eastern Economic Review 162 (1999): 38-40. UMI-ProQuest Direct. [Online] [April 13, 1999].

[37] Kanehisa, H., M. Kondo, S. Ikegawa, and T. Fukunaga. (1997). "Characteristics of body composition and muscle strength in college sumo wrestlers." <u>International Journal of Sports Medicine</u> 18 (1997): 510-515.

[37] Nishizawa, T., I. Akaoka, Y. Nishida, Y. Kawaguchi, E. Hayashi, and T. Yashimura. "Some factor related to obesity in the Japanese sumo wrestler." <u>The American Journal of Clinical Nutrition</u> 29 (1976): 1167-1174.

[38] Nishizawa, T., I. Akaoka, Y. Nishida, Y. Kawaguchi, E. Hayashi, and T. Yashimura. "Some factor related to obesity in the Japanese sumo wrestler." <u>The American Journal of Clinical Nutrition</u> 29 (1976): 1167-1174.

The Low Carb Myth by Champion Brad Schoenfeld

[39] Farnsworth E., et al. "Effect of a high-protein, energy-restricted diet on body composition, glycemic control, and lipid concentrations in overweight and obese hyperinsulinemic men and women." <u>American Journal of Clinical Nutrition</u> 78(1) (2003 Jul): 31-39.

[40] Peterson C.M., et al. "Randomized crossover study of 40% vs. 55% carbohydrate weight loss strategies in women with previous gestational diabetes mellitus and non-diabetic women of 130-200% ideal body weight." Journal of the American College of Nutrition 14(4) (1995 Aug): 369-375.

[41] Bravata T.M., et al. "Efficacy and safety of low-carbohydrate diets: a systematic review." Journal of the American Medical Association 289(14) (2003 Apr 9): 1837-1850. Review.

[42] Luscombe N.D., et al. "Effect of a high-protein, energy-restricted diet on weight loss and energy expenditure after weight stabilization in hyperinsulinemic subjects." International Journal of Obesity Related Metabolic Disorders 27(5) (2003 May): 582-590.

[43] Golay A., et al. "Similar weight loss with low- or high-carbohydrate diets." American Journal of Clinical Nutrition 63(2) (1996 Feb): 174-178.

[44] Baba N.H., et al. "High protein vs high carbohydrate hypoenergetic diet for the treatment of obese hyperinsulinemic subjects." International Journal of Obesity Related Metabolic Disorders 23(11) (1999 Nov): 1202-1206.

[45] Smith G.P., et al. "Are gut peptides a new class of anorectic agents?" American Journal of Clinical Nutriition 55 (1 Suppl) (1992 Jan): 283S-285S. Review.

[46] Samaha F.F., et al. "A low-carbohydrate as compared with a low-fat diet in severe obesity." New England Journal of Medicine 348(21) (2003 May 22): 2074-2081.

[47] Riegler, E. "Weight reduction by a high protein, low carbohydrate diet." Med Klin 71(24) (1976 Jun 11): 1051-1056.

[48] Pirozzo S., et al. "Should we recommend low-fat diets for obesity?" Obesity Review 4(2) (2003 May): 83-90. Review.

Tennis Fitness, Anyone? by Champion Robert L. Selders, Jr.

Baechle, T.R. and R.W. Earle. Essentials of Strength and Conditioning, 2nd edition. Champaign, IL: Human Kinetics, 2000.

Knudson, D., K. Bennett, R. Corn, D. Leick, and C. Smith. "Acute Effects of Stretching Are Not Evident in the Kinematics of the Vertical Jump." Journal of Strength and Conditioning Research 15 (1) (2001): 98-101.

National Academy of Sports Medicine. Optimum Performance Training for the Performance Enhancement Specialist: Home Study Course Manual. Calabasas, CA: National Academy of Sports Medicine, 2002.

Rotert, P., and T.S. Ellenbecker. Complete Conditioning for Tennis. Champaign, IL: Human Kinetics, 1998.

My Aching Back by Champion Katie Mital

[49] American Council on Exercise. <u>Clinical Exercise Specialist Manual</u>. San Diego, CA: American Council on Exercise, 1999.

Illustrations by Tom Mital.

Too Old? by Doug Carlyle

[50] Leif, Alex, M.D. "The Magic Anti-Aging Bullet: Exercise." <u>Personal Training Associates</u>. http://www.pta1.com/index.html?magic_bullet.html.

Overtraining: When Exercise Becomes Too Much of a Good Thing by Champion Sandy Rusch

Raglin, Jack, M.D. "Exercise Addiction and Overtraining." Seminar presented at Fitness Mania, Sara's City Workout. Chicago, IL: Nov 2003.

Rest and Recovery from Exercise by Champion Jason Brice

[51] Kurz, T. <u>Science of Sports Training: How to Plan and Control Training for Peak Performance</u>, Island Pond, VT: Stadion Publishing Company, 2001.

[52] Siff, M.C. and M. Yessis, eds. <u>Sports Restoration and Massage.</u> School of Mechanical Engineering, University of Witwatersrand, South Africa.

Fat Burning Secrets for Women by Champion Kelli Calabrese

[53] Nelson, M. et al. "Effects of high-intensity strength training on multiple risk factors for osteoporotic fractures." <u>Journal of the American Medical Association</u> 272 (1994): 1909-1914.

[54] Ballor, D. and E. Poehlman. "Exercise training enhances fat free mass preservation during diet-induced weight loss: a meta analytic finding." <u>International Journal of Obesity</u> 18 (1994): 35-40.

[55] Campbell, W. et al. "Increased energy requirements and changes in body composition with resistance training in older adults." <u>American Journal of Clinical Nutrition</u>, 60 (1994): 167-175.

Recommended web sites:

Is A Health Club Right For Me? by Champion Joe Stankowski

www.thepowerofchampions.com
www.absolutefitnessUSA.com
www.ihrsa.org
www.dolfzine.com
www.ideafit.com
www.acefitness.org
www.nasm.org

Be Your Own Fitness Coach by Champion Tony Rodriguez

www.wellcoaches.com

Index

S

T

U

V

visualization 62, 66

W

walking buddy 219
warm up 103
water 161, 182
weight-bearing exercise 91
Wolff's Law 76
wrist girth 87

Y

yo-yo effect 257
yoga 220
"Yucant" Bug 6